Cleanroom Technology

Cleanroom Technology

Fundamentals of Design, Testing and Operation

W. Whyte
University of Glasgow, UK

JOHN WILEY & SONS, LTD
Chichester • New York • Weinheim • Brisbane • Singapore • Toronto

Published by John Wiley & Sons Ltd,
Baffins Lane, Chichester,
West Sussex PO19 1UD, England
National 01243 779777
International (+44) 1243 779777

e-mail (for order and customer service enquiries):
cs-books@wiley.co.uk

Visit our Home Page on http://www.wiley.co.uk or
http://www.wiley.com

Other Wiley Editorial Offices

John Wiley & Sons, Inc., 605 Third Avenue,
New York, NY 10158-0012, USA

WILEY-VCH Verlag GmbH, Pappelallee 3,
D-69469 Weinheim, Germany

Jacaranda Wiley Ltd, 33 Park Road, Milton,
Queensland 4064, Australia

John Wiley & Sons (Asia) Pte Ltd, 2 Clementi Loop #02-01,
Jin Xing Distripark, Singapore 129809

John Wiley & Sons (Canada) Ltd, 22 Worcester Road,
Rexdale, Ontario M9W 1L1, Canada

British Library Cataloguing in Publication Data

A catalogue record for this book is available from the British Library

ISBN 0 471 86842 6

Produced from computer files supplied by the author
Printed and bound in Great Britain by Biddles Ltd, Guildford and King's Lynn
This book is printed on acid-free paper responsibly manufactured from sustainable forestry, in which at least two trees are planted for each one used for paper production.

Contents

Preface

The dirt and bacterial-free conditions provided by cleanrooms are essential for much of modern manufacturing industry. Without clean conditions, products get contaminated and either malfunction or become hazardous to people. In recent years there has been a considerable increase in the number of cleanrooms. They are now used for the manufacture of items used in computers, cars, aeroplanes, spacecraft, televisions, disc players and many other electronic and mechanical devices, as well as the manufacture of medicines, medical devices and convenience foods. This rapid increase in the use of cleanrooms has created a demand for good quality information about cleanrooms that is free from the 'hype' of sales and marketing jargon. Information is also required to teach production personnel about their working environment, and how to conduct themselves within the cleanroom to minimise contamination.

Cleanroom technology can be divided into three parts: design, testing and operation. Cleanrooms have to be first designed and constructed; they then have to be tested to ensure they achieve their design specification and continue to do so; finally they have to be operated in such a way as to minimise contamination. This book covers, in a holistic way, these three main facets of cleanroom technology.

This book has been written using the principals generally accepted within cleanroom industries. However, I have found many areas where no sound advice exists and have had to develop guidance using my knowledge and experience. Because of this, I have tried wherever possible to give the scientific reasons for the contamination control measures suggested, so that the worth of my opinions may be judged. However, many of the principals are one man's opinion, and this should be borne in mind.

This book is intended for anyone involved with cleanrooms who wishes an overview of the fundamentals of cleanroom design, testing and operation. However, it is inevitable that with my teaching background I would wish to help those who instruct, or are about to instruct, the subject of 'Cleanroom Technology' either at college, or to their cleanroom personnel. I hope the information given in this book is helpful in achieving these requirements.

Acknowledgements

During my many years of involvement with cleanrooms I have been fortunate to meet many of the people who pioneered and developed cleanroom technology. Many of them I now consider as friends. From these people I received information that assisted me during my career; it is from my career experience that this book has been written. It would be impossible to name all of these people, and they must forgive me if they see an idea that they know was theirs. I must confine myself to acknowledging the help of those people who directly contributed to this book. This contribution has been in the nature of: being a co-author of an article that I have used when writing this book; reading and commenting on a chapter; helping in producing photographs. These people are (in alphabetical order) Neil Bell, Chuck Bernt, Roger Diener, Gordon Farquharson, Gordon King, Lynn Morrison, Bob Peck, Martin Reeves, Hal Smith and Neil Stephenson. I should also like to acknowledge the support of the Scottish Society for Contamination Control.

The photographs on the cover of this book are reproduced by permission of Aberdeen City Council, Library and Information Service, Pentagon Technology, Analog Devices and Evanite Fiber Corporation. The permission to use other photographs, tables and drawings used within the book is acknowledged at the end of each chapter. Isabelle Lawson produced most of the drawings in this book, and Barbara McLeod read and commented on the script.

1

Introduction

1.1 What is a Cleanroom?

It is clear that a cleanroom is a room that is clean. However, a cleanroom now has a special meaning and it is defined in the International Organization for Standarization (ISO) standard 14644-1 as:

> *A room in which the concentration of airborne particles is controlled, and which is constructed and used in a manner to minimise the introduction, generation, and retention of particles inside the room and in which other relevant parameters, e.g. temperature, humidity, and pressure, are controlled as necessary.*

The first two thirds of the definition is, in essence, what a cleanroom is. It is a room that minimises the introduction, generation and retention of particles. This is achieved, firstly, by supplying it with exceptionally large quantities of air that has been filtered with high efficiency filters. This air is used to (1) dilute and remove the particles and bacteria dispersed from personnel and machinery within the room and, (2) to pressurise the room and ensure that no dirty air flows into the cleanroom. Secondly, a cleanroom is built with materials that do not generate particles and can be easily cleaned. Finally, cleanroom personnel use clothing that envelops them and minimises their dispersion of particles and micro-organisms. These and other similar measures that minimise the introduction, generation and retention of contamination in a cleanroom are discussed in this book. Cleanrooms can also control the temperature, humidity, sound, lighting, and vibration. However, these parameters are not exclusive to cleanrooms, and are therefore not discussed in any detail in this book.

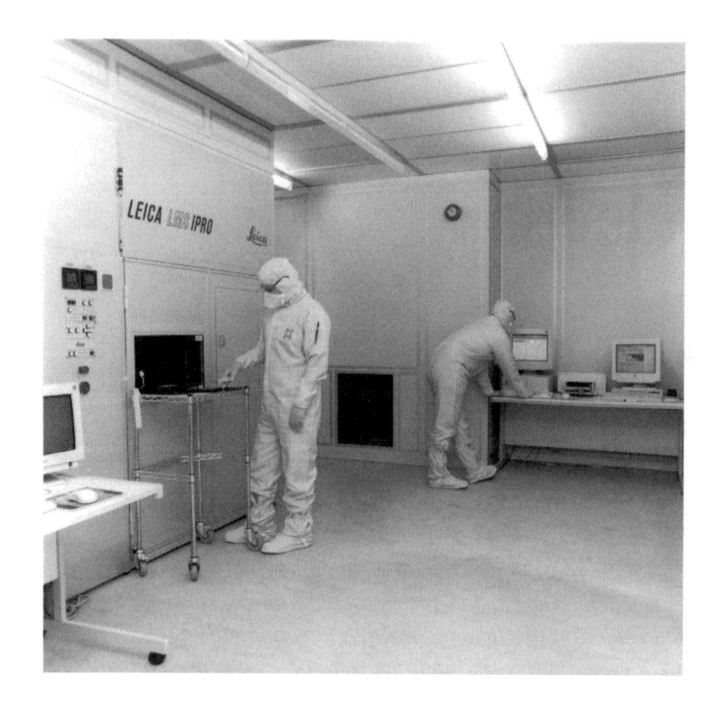

Figure 1.1 A cleanroom with personnel wearing special cleanroom clothing.

1.2 The Need for Cleanrooms

The cleanroom is a modern phenomenon. Although the roots of cleanroom design and management go back for more than 100 years and are rooted in the control of infection in hospitals, the need for a clean environment for industrial manufacturing is a requirement of modern society. Cleanrooms are needed because people, production machinery and the building structure generate contamination. As will be discussed later in this book, people and machinery produce millions of particles, and conventional building materials can easily break up. A cleanroom controls this dispersion and allows manufacturing to be carried out in a clean environment.

The uses of cleanrooms are diverse; shown in Table 1.1 is a selection of products that are now being made in cleanrooms.

Table 1.1 Some cleanroom applications

Industry	Product
Electronics	Computers, TV-tubes, flat screens
Semiconductor	Production of integrated circuits used in computer memory and control
Micromechanics	Gyroscopes, miniature bearings, compact-disc players
Optics	Lenses, photographic film, laser equipment

Biotechnology	Antibiotic production, genetic engineering
Pharmacy	Sterile pharmaceuticals, sterile disposables
Medical Devices	Heart valves, cardiac by-pass systems
Food and Drink	Brewery production, unsterilized food and drink

It may be seen in Table 1.1 that cleanroom applications can be broadly divided into two. In the top section of Table 1.1 are those industries where dust particles are a problem, and their presence, even in sub-micrometre size, may prevent a product functioning, or reduce its useful life.

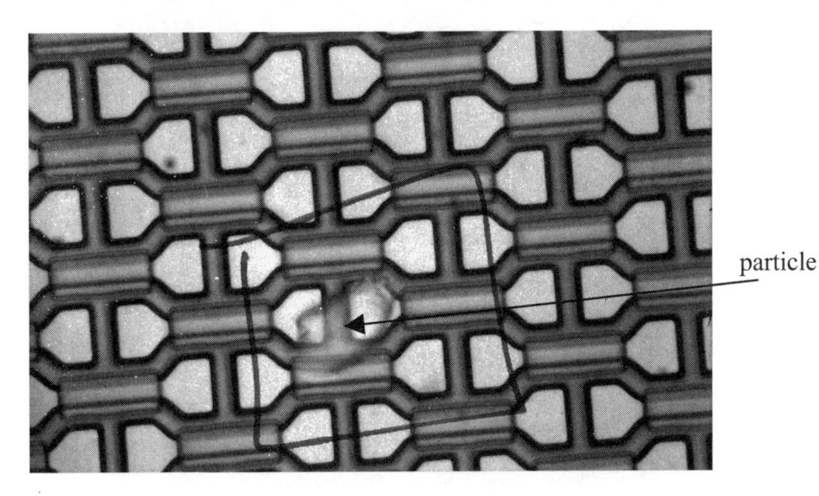

Figure 1.2 Contaminating particle on a semiconductor

A major user of cleanrooms is the semiconductor fabrication industry, where processors are produced for use in computers, cars and other machines. Figure 1.2 shows a photomicrograph of a semiconductor with a particle on it. Such particles can cause an electrical short and ruin the semiconductor. To minimise contamination problems, semiconductors are manufactured in cleanrooms with very high standards of cleanliness.

The bottom section of Table 1.1 shows manufacturers who require the absence of micro-organisms, as their growth in a product (or in a hospital patient) could lead to human infection. The healthcare industry is a major user of cleanrooms, as micro-organisms or dirt must not be injected or infused into patients through their products. Hospital operating rooms also use cleanroom technology to minimise wound infection (Figure 1.3).

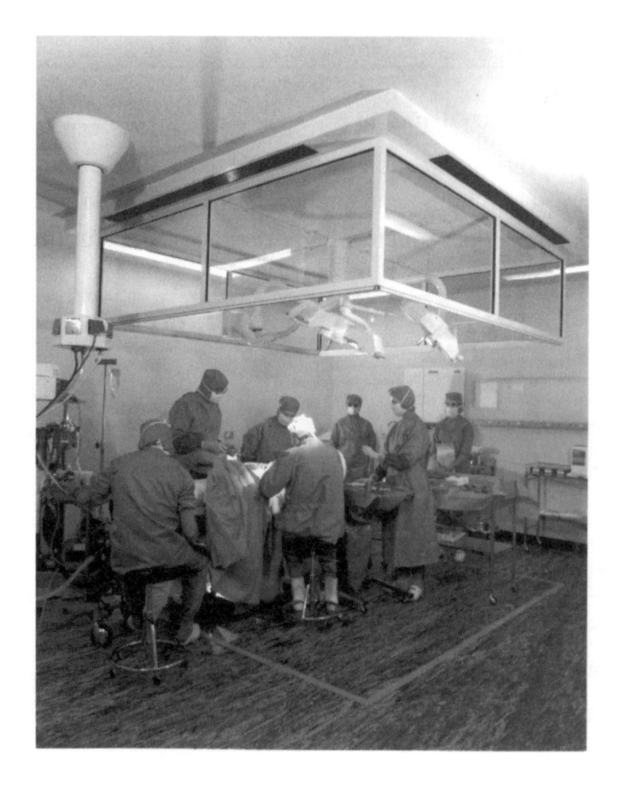

Figure 1.3 Unidirectional flow system in an operating room

It may also be seen from Table 1.1 that many of the examples are recent innovations and this list will certainly be added to in the future, there being a considerable and expanding demand for these type of rooms.

1.3 Types of Cleanrooms

Cleanrooms have evolved into two major types and they are differentiated by their method of ventilation. These are *turbulently ventilated* and *unidirectional flow cleanrooms*. Turbulently ventilated cleanrooms are also known as 'nonunidirectional'. Unidirectional flow cleanrooms were originally known as 'laminar flow' cleanrooms. The unidirectional type of cleanroom uses very much more air than the turbulently ventilated type, and gives superior cleanliness.

The two major types of cleanroom are shown diagrammatically in Figures 1.4 and 1.5. Figure 1.4 shows a turbulently ventilated room receiving clean filtered air through air diffusers in the ceiling. This air mixes with the room air and removes airborne contamination through air extracts at the bottom of the walls.

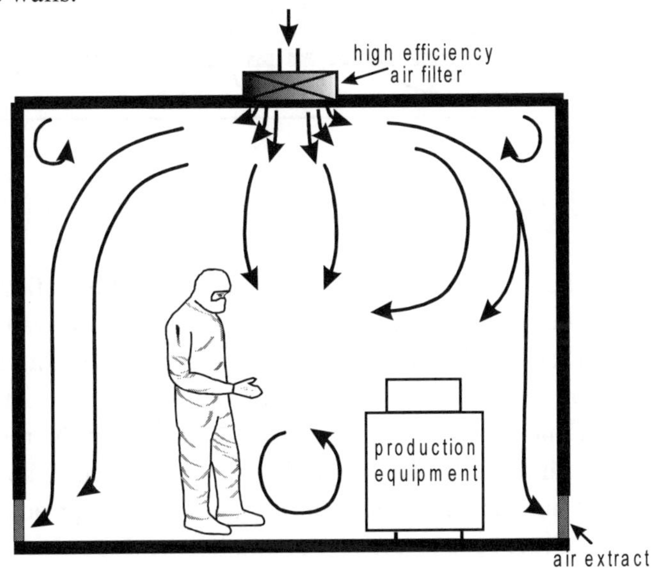

Figure 1.4 Conventionally ventilated type of cleanroom

The air changes are normally equal to, or greater than, 20 per hour, this being much greater than that used in ordinary rooms, such as in offices. In this style of cleanroom, the contamination generated by people and machinery is mixed and diluted with the supply air and then removed.

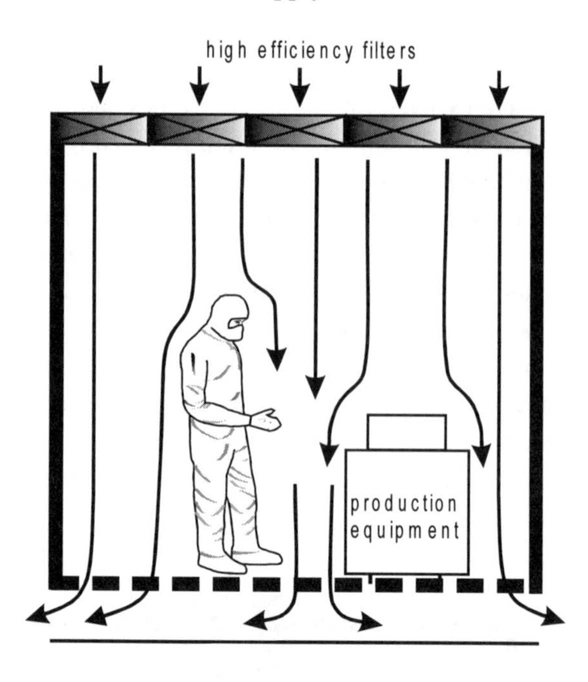

Figure 1.5 Unidirectional flow type of cleanroom

Figure 1.5 shows the basic principles of a unidirectional flow room. High efficiency filters are installed across a whole ceiling (or wall in some systems) and these supply air. This air sweeps across the room in a unidirectional way at a speed of around 0.4 m/s (80 ft/min) and exits through the floor, thus removing the airborne contamination from the room. This system uses much more air than the turbulently ventilated cleanroom but, because of the directed air movement, it minimises the spread of contamination about the room and sweeps it out through the floor.

Clean air devices, such as unidirectional benches or isolators, are used in both turbulently and unidirectional ventilated cleanrooms. These machines will give a localised supply of filtered air and enhanced air conditions where required, e.g. at the area where the product is open to contamination.

1.5 What is Cleanroom Technology?

As can be seen in Figure 1.6, cleanroom technology can be divided into three broad areas. These areas can also be seen to parallel the use of the technology as the cleanroom user moves from firstly deciding to purchase a room to finally operating it.

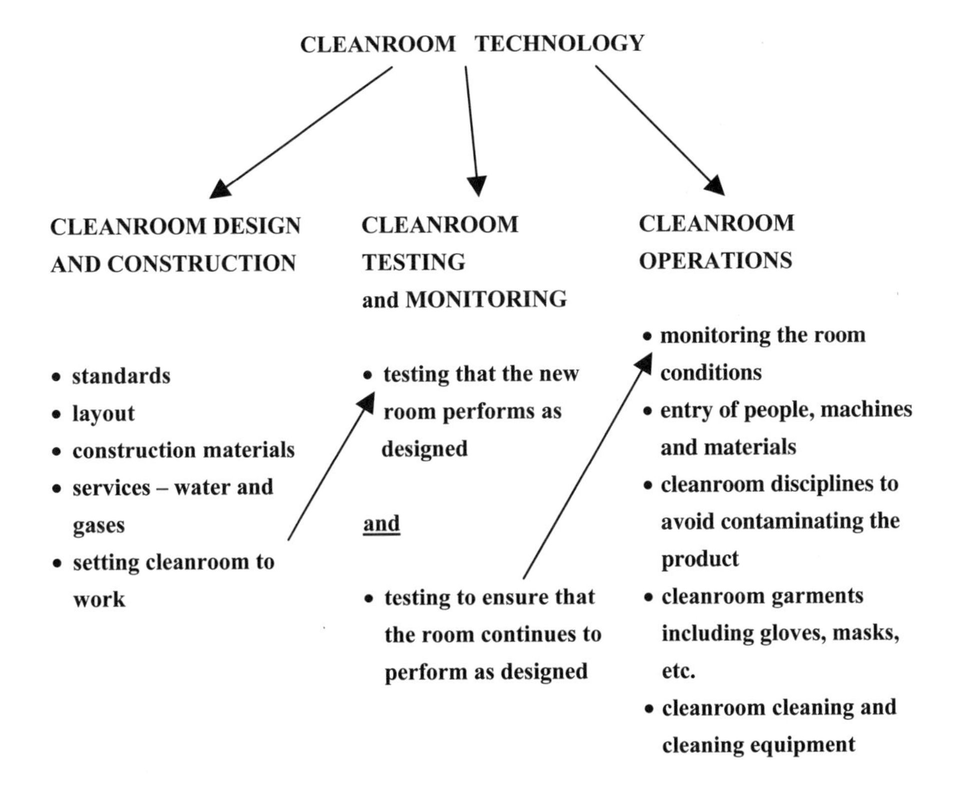

Figure 1.6 Various parts of cleanroom technology and their interconnections

Firstly, it is necessary to *design and construct* the room. To do this one must consider (1) the design standards that should be used, (2) what design layout and construction materials can be used, and (3) how services should be supplied to the cleanroom.

Secondly, after the cleanroom has been installed and working, it must be *tested* to check that it conforms to the stipulated design. During the life of the cleanroom, the room must also be *monitored* to ensure that it continually achieves the standards that are required.

Finally, it is necessary to *operate* the cleanroom correctly so that the manufactured products are not contaminated. This requires that the entry of people and materials, the garment selection, cleanroom disciplines and the cleaning of the room are all correctly carried out.

These fundamental elements of Cleanroom Technology are covered in this book.

Acknowledgements

Figure 1.1 is reproduced by permission of Compugraphics and M+W Pearce. Figure 1.3 is reproduced by permission of Fishers Services.

2

The History of Cleanrooms

2.1 The Early Years

It is clear that the first cleanrooms were in hospitals. Lord Lister's contribution to history was his realisation that bacteria caused surgical wound infection. He thought that the elimination of bacteria from the operating room should prevent infection. This was the scientific basis for the first cleanrooms.

In the 1860s, Lister dramatically reduced infection in his operating room at the Royal Infirmary, Glasgow by use of an antiseptic solution (carbolic acid) that killed bacteria. He used this on the instruments, the wound and the surgeon's hands, and he attempted to prevent airborne infection by spraying it into the air.

Shown in Figure 2.1 is a photograph taken in 1889 of a group of surgeons from the Aberdeen Royal Infirmary in Scotland using Lister's spray, which sprayed carbolic acid into the air of an operating room. This photograph is interesting from several points of view. Lister's spray is of historical interest, although it probably did little to reduce airborne bacteria. Also to be seen is the surgeon Ogston, who is the third figure from the right. He was the discoverer of the bacteria *Staphylococcus aureus*, an important cause of wound sepsis, then and now.

It is interesting to observe the accepted mode of dress at that time. Although this photograph is probably posed, operations at that time were carried out without the protection of sterile (or even clean) clothing. The surgeon would often operate wearing an old frock coat contaminated with bloody pus and bacteria. He might wear an apron or gown, but this would be used to protect him from blood and not meant to protect the patient from his bacteria.

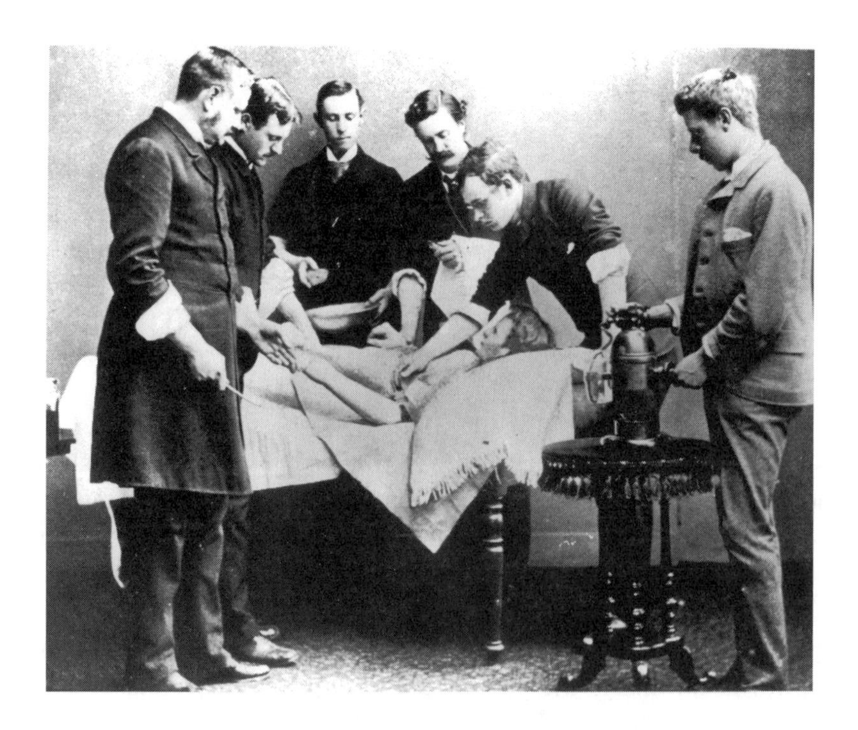

Figure 2.1 A group of surgeons with the Lister steam spray.

A photograph taken in the Royal Infirmary, Edinburgh, Scotland in the 1890s (Figure 2.2) shows a number of aspects of surgery that will interest those working in modern cleanrooms. The gas lamp seen in the top left-hand side of the picture confirms the age of the photograph, as do many other aspects.

The surgeons can be seen to be wearing gowns, but not gloves, hats or masks. In the background of the operating rooms is a gallery where the medical students would crowd in to see the operation without consideration of the bacteria they dispersed; the gallery is the reason that operating rooms are still called operating 'theatres' in many parts of the world. The floor is exposed wooden flooring, and the sinks, buckets and exposed pipes reflect a bygone age where little was known of contamination control.

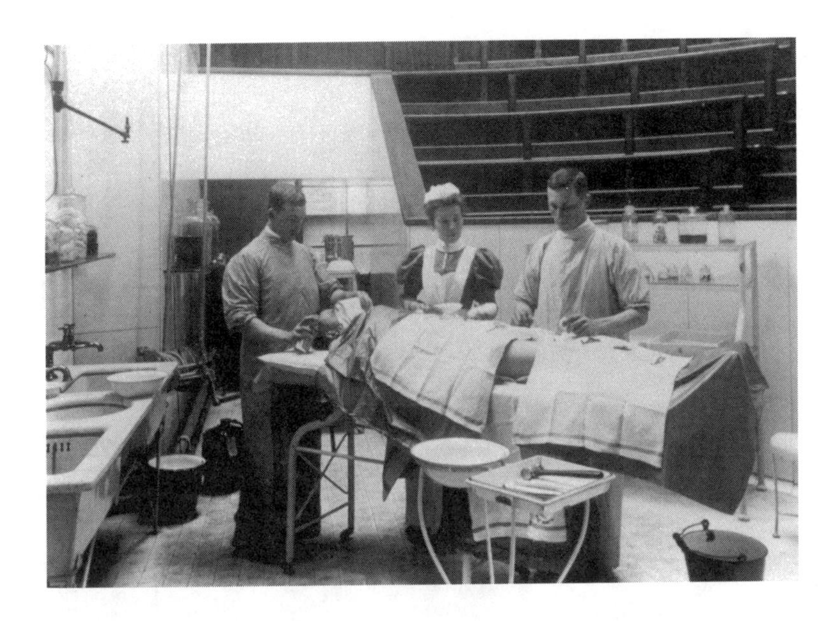

Figure 2.2 An operating room in the late 1890s.

Lord Lister's reduction of wound sepsis was by an *antiseptic* method, as he used a disinfectant to kill the bacteria on bandages, the hands of the surgeon and in the operating room environment. One of his former assistants, Sir William Macewan, who succeeded Lister as Professor of Surgery at the University of Glasgow, along with other surgeons in Germany and the USA, developed Lister's techniques into the field of *aseptic* techniques. By aseptic means they sought not to kill bacteria that entered the wound, but to prevent them from getting there. Boiling of instruments and bandages was introduced and the surgeons and nurses ensured their hands were rigorously 'scrubbed' to remove bacteria. By the year 1900, surgical gloves, masks and gowns had been introduced. These could be steam sterilised before an operation, although at a lower temperature and pressure than used today. These methods were the basis of cleanroom techniques used today.

Shown in Figure 2.3 is an operating room in the Royal Infirmary, Edinburgh, photographed around 1907. The contrast to the photograph in Figure 2.2 is noticeable. Electricity has been installed, but of more interest is the fact that the surgeon can be seen to wear gloves and a facemask. The face-

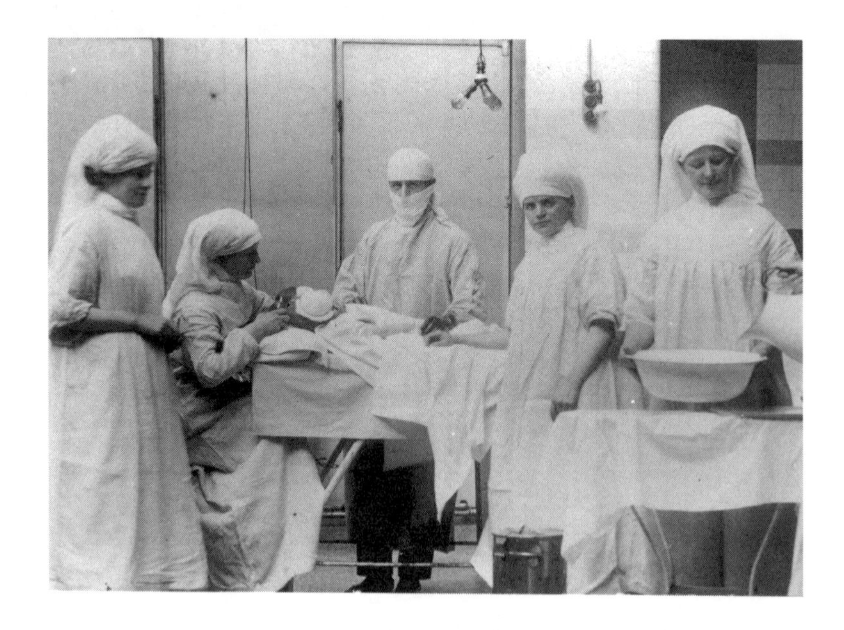

Figure 2.3 Operating room in 1907 showing aseptic precautions

mask is below his nose, as it was not till the end of the 1930s that it was appreciated that it should go over the nose. There is also a terrazzo-type floor and tiled walls to facilitate disinfection and cleaning.

2.2 Ventilated Operating Rooms

Although the operating rooms of yesteryear had contamination control methods that were similar to modern cleanrooms, an important omission was positive ventilation with filtered air. Artificial ventilation was rarely used in hospitals in temperate climates until the 1940s, and where ventilation was used it was more for comfort than contamination control. It was only after the end of the Second World War (1945) that ventilation in hospitals was clearly advocated for contamination control. The problems of airborne infection of people in crowded situations that occurred in wartime, e.g. submarines, air raid shelters and army barracks, were studied. Microbiological warfare required the airborne dispersion of micro-organisms and this was also studied. The airborne bacterial sampler was invented, and the ventilation of rooms and aerodynamics of particles were all studied during the Second World War.

By the early 1960s, most of the principles that dictate the performance of turbulently ventilated rooms were known. Also established was the fact that people were the source of airborne bacteria, these being dispersed on rafts of skin, and that open-weave cotton garments did little to prevent this dispersion; tightly woven fabrics were required.

In 1960 Blowers and Crew attempted to obtain a downward 'piston' of air (unidirectional flow, although they did not call it that) from an air diffuser fitted over the entire ceiling in an operating room in Middlesborough in England. Unfortunately, because of the thermal air currents from people and the operating room lamp, as well as movement of people, the low air velocity was disrupted; this made it impossible to achieve good unidirectional airflow. This was the situation when Professor Sir John Charnley (with assistance from Howorth Air Conditioning) decided to improve the ventilation in his operating room at Wrightington Hospital near Manchester in England.

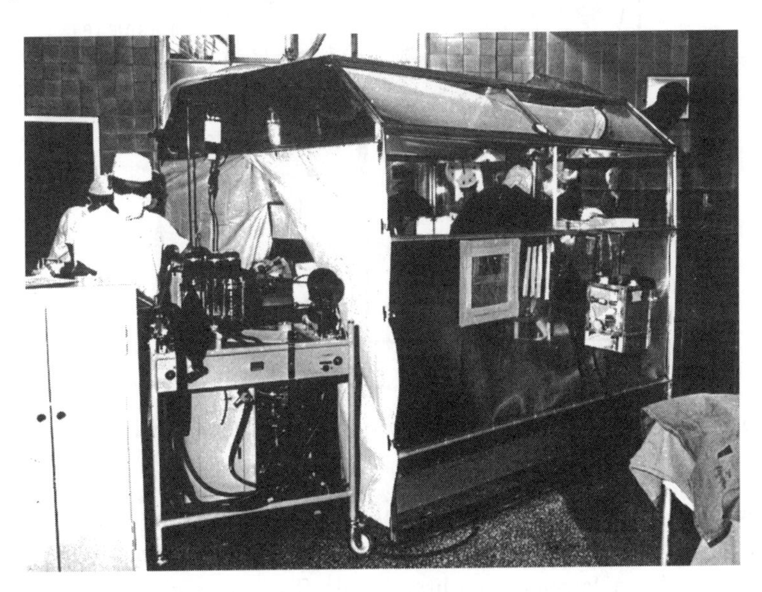

Figure 2.4 The Charnley-Howorth 'greenhouse'

Charnley was a pioneer of hip replacement surgery. He devised an operation to replace a diseased joint with an artificial plastic and metal one. His initial operations gave a sepsis rate in the region of 10%. This was a major problem, and so he initiated a number of preventative measures. Using the knowledge that existed at the time (1961), Howorth and he attempted to perfect the 'piston effect' of a downward flow of air. Instead of using the whole of the operating room ceiling (as Blowers and Crew had done) they restricted it to a small area and hence improved the downward flow of air. They used a 7ft × 7ft-area 'greenhouse' placed within the operating room. This is shown in Figure 2.4.

Figure 2.5 shows the diagram Charnley published of the airflow in the system; it can be seen that reasonable downward unidirectional flow was achieved.

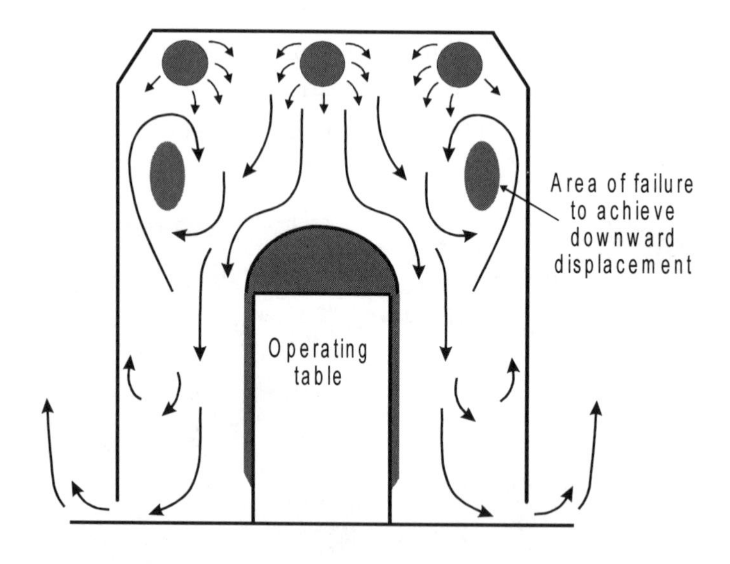

Figure 2.5 Section through Charnley's original system showing the airflow

Charnley and Howorth Air Conditioning increased the air supply volume and then incorporated design improvements using the knowledge gained from the work on laminar (unidirectional) flow systems in the USA and elsewhere. He found that the improvements in his operating room, and in the fabric and design of clothing substantially reduced airborne bacteria. These reductions were paralleled with reductions in deep hip infection. These were reduced from about 10% in 1959, when his operating room conditions were poor, to less than 1.0% by 1970 when all his improvements were complete. The Medical Research Council of the United Kingdom confirmed in the 1980s that the use of unidirectional flow enclosures with occlusive clothing would reduce the joint sepsis to one quarter of that found in turbulently ventilated operating rooms.

2.3 Early Industrial Cleanrooms

In engineering industries, similar advances were being made. The development of the first cleanrooms for industrial manufacturing started during the Second World War, this was mainly in an attempt to improve the quality and reliability of instrumentation used in guns, tanks and aircraft. It was realised that the cleanliness of the production environment had to be improved, or items such as bombsights would malfunction. However, it was assumed that cleanrooms were kept clean like people's homes. Surfaces like stainless steel, which did not generate particles, were used and kept clean. It was not appreciated that the airborne dispersion of large quantities of particles by machines and people should be minimised by supplying large quantities of clean air. For example, the dominant idea in a pharmaceutical production room was that it had to be kept free of micro-organisms by the use of copious quantities of disinfectants. The walls were made suitable for this purpose often being tiled, and the floor would be a terrazzo-type having a gully and drains to remove the disinfectant. Ventilation was very basic, there being few air changes per hour, and there was little in the way of air movement control within the room, or between the production area and outside areas. Personnel were dressed in cotton clothing similar to that used in the operating rooms of that era, and clothes changing areas, if they existed, were very basic.

The use of nuclear fission, as well as the biological and chemical warfare research carried out during the 1939–1945 Second World War, were the driving forces for the production of High Efficiency Particulate Air (HEPA) filters necessary to contain the dangerous microbial or radioactive contaminants. Their availability allowed cleanrooms to be supplied with very clean air, and low levels of airborne contamination to be achieved.

Rooms with large volumes of well-filtered air supplied by ceiling diffusers were built between 1955 and the early 1960s. In the early 1950s the Western Electric Company in Winston-Salem, NC, USA was having a major problem in manufacturing missile gyroscopes. About 99 out of 100 gyroscopes were being rejected, the problem being identified as dust. It was decided that a 'dust free' production room should be built and this was designed by the AC Corporation and completed in 1955. Figure 2.6 shows the room soon after production started.

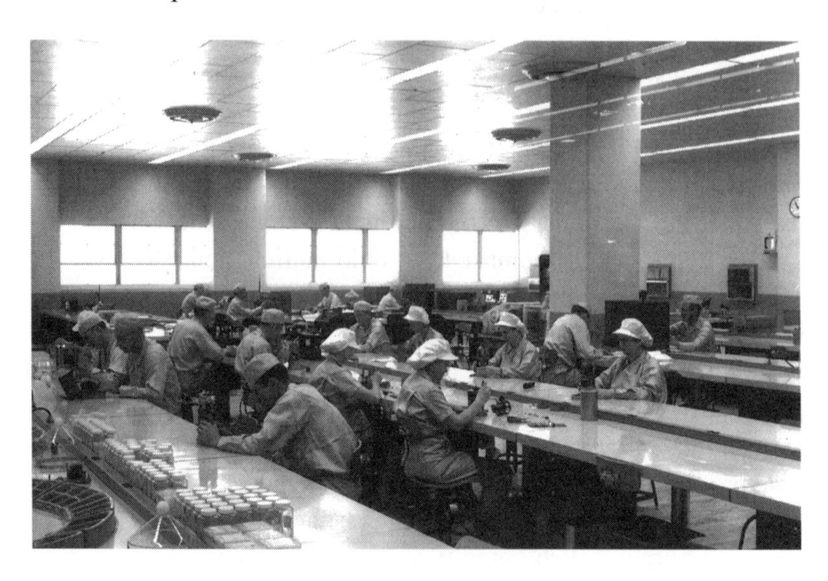

Figure 2.6 Gyroscope production room at Western Electric

This may be the first production cleanroom built that recognised all of the basic requirements of a cleanroom. Personnel wore synthetic fabric clothing with a cap; they also had a locker room for changing clothes. Construction materials were chosen for ease of cleaning and to minimise the production of particles. Cracks and corners were minimised and the vinyl-covered floors were coved onto the wall and the lighting was flush-mounted to minimise dust accumulation. As can be seen in the back right-hand side of the photograph, pass-through windows were used. The air-conditioned supply was filtered through 'absolute' filters that were capable of removing 99.95% of 0.3 μm particles, and the room was positively pressurised.

2.4 Unidirectional Flow Cleanrooms

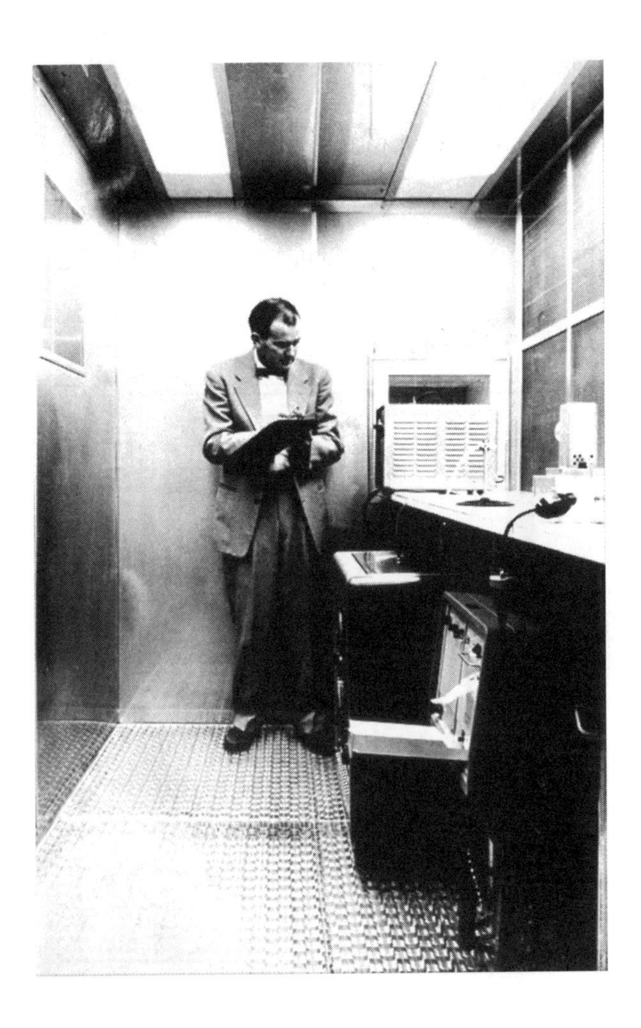

Figure 2.7 Willis Whitfield in his original laminar flow room

The watershed in the history of cleanrooms was the invention, in 1961, of the 'unidirectional' or 'laminar flow' concept of ventilation at the Sandia Laboratories, Albuquerque, New Mexico, USA. This was a team effort, but it is to Willis Whitfield that the main credit goes. Shown in Figure 2.7 is a photograph of him in his original room.

The room was small, being 6 ft wide by 10 ft long by 7 ft high (1.8 m × 3 m × 2.1 m). Instead of the air being supplied by ceiling diffusers and moving about the room in a random way, it was supplied by a bank of HEPA filters. This ensured that air moved in a unidirectional way from the filters across the room and out through the floor grilles. Shown in Figure 2.8 is a cross-sectional drawing of the original unidirectional airflow room. It may be seen that anyone working at the bench in the room should not contaminate anything in front of them, as their contamination would be swept away.

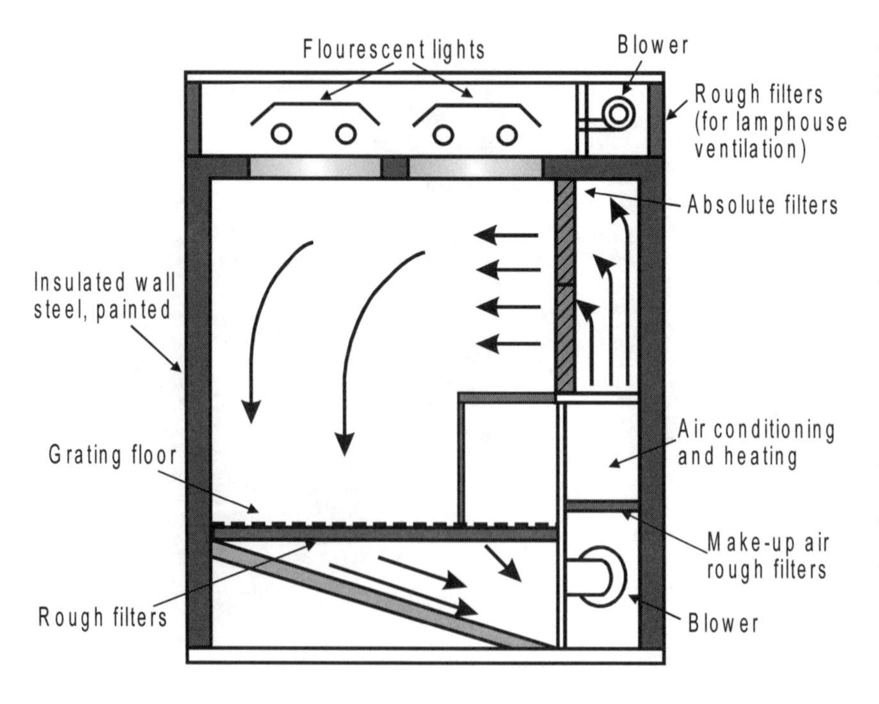

Figure 2.8 A cross-section of the original unidirectional cleanroom

The invention at Sandia was publicised in *Time* magazine of April 13th 1962, and this article created a great deal of interest. The article was as follows:

'Mr Clean

Scientists at the Sandia Corp. in Albuquerque, where nuclear weapons are designed and assembled, have a passion for cleanliness. They have to. As weapons components are made smaller and still smaller, the presence of a single particle of dust can make larger and still larger trouble. The strictest housekeeper in all Sandia is Texas-born Physicist Willis J. Whitfield, creator of the Whitfield Ultra-Clean Room. "I thought about dust particles," he says with a slight drawl. "Where are these rascals generated? Where do they go?" Once he answered his own questions Physicist Whitfield decided that conventional industrial clean rooms are wrong in principle.

The usual system in clean rooms, which are necessary for an ever-increasing number of industrial operations, is to keep dust particles from being released. Smoking is forbidden; so are ordinary pencils, which give off graphite particles. People who work in the clean rooms are "packaged" in special boots, hoods and coveralls and are vacuum-cleaned before they enter. The rooms themselves are vacuumed continually. But despite all these precautions each cubic foot of their air still contains at least 1,000,000 dust particles that are .3 microns (.000012 in.) or larger in diameter. This is a vast improvement over ordinary air, but Whitfield was sure he could do better. Abandoning the idea of keeping dust particles from being generated, he decided to remove them as soon as they appear.

The Whitfield Ultra-Clean Room looks like a small metal house trailer without wheels. Its floor is metal grating. It is lined with stainless steel, and along one wall the workbench faces a 4 ft by 10 ft bank of "absolute filters" that remove all particles above .3 microns from a slow stream of air. Most clean rooms use their filters simply to clean up incoming air. Whitfield's trick is to make the clean air from the filters keep the room clean. It flows at 1 mph (a very faint breeze) across the workbench and past the people working at it. Workmen can dress in ordinary clothes and smoke if they desire. Dandruff, tobacco smoke, pencil dust and any other particles generated are carried away by the clean air, whisked down through the grating floor, and discharged outdoors. Every six seconds the room gets a change of ultra-clean air. No particles get a chance to circulate, and as a result, Physicist Whitfield's room is at least 1,000 times as clean as the cleanest of its competitor'.

The concept of unidirectional flow cleanroom ventilation was very quickly adopted by a large variety of industries, as high quality cleanrooms were urgently required.

Acknowledgements

Figure 2.1 is reproduced by permission of Aberdeen City Council, Library and Information Services. Figure 2.2 and Figures 2.3 are reproduced by permission of Lothian Health Services Archive, Edinburgh University Library. Figure 2.4 is reproduced by permission of Howorth Airtech Ltd. Figure 2.5 is reproduced by permission of British Journal of Surgery. The article 'Mr Clean' is reproduced by permission of Time Inc.

3

Cleanroom classification standards

3.1 The History

It can be argued, with justification, that the first standard written for cleanrooms was published by the American Airforce on March 1961 and known as Technical Manual (T.O.) 00-25-203. This considered cleanroom design and airborne particle standards, as well as operating procedures such as: entry procedures; clothing; restriction of certain articles; cleaning of materials; procedures for cleaning the room. However, the standard that had the most influence on the design and operation of cleanrooms, and is the basis of most world cleanroom standards, including ISO standard 14644-1, was Federal Standard 209.

The Sandia Corporation team that invented the unidirectional concept, aided by others from the USA military, industry and governmental agencies, produced the first Federal Standard 209 in 1963. This standard discussed both conventional and unidirectional cleanrooms. In the standard there is the first suggestion of measuring particles of ≥ 0.5μm by means of optical particle counters; these instruments had just become commercially available. It often asked why 0.5 μm was adopted as the standard size on which the Federal Standard was based. The answer is that it was the 'art of the achievable', as this was the smallest size that was easily measured by the particle counters available at that time.

It has been asked why 90 ft/min was suggested in the Federal Standard 209 as the velocity to be used in unidirectional flow cleanrooms. It has been said that this was the velocity theoretically calculated to remove a particle dropped in front of the supply filter in the first laminar flow room at Sandia Corporation. An alternative opinion given was that the only air supply fan available to Willis Whitfield gave this air velocity. I have discussed this with Willis Whitfield who said that the fan was capable of giving velocities of between 50 ft/min and 200 ft/min. When the room was run at high velocities, it was very noisy and expensive to maintain. When run at 50 ft/min, and with only one person in it, it was possible to obtain good particle counts. However, if several people were in the room, a velocity of about 90 ft/min to 100 ft/min was required to control the particle contamination. As he and his team were under pressure to produce data for the design of unidirectional cleanrooms, and little time was available for a thorough scientific evaluation, this velocity was adopted.

Cleanroom standards have been written to cater for the needs of the expanded cleanroom industry. These are discussed below.

3.2 The Basis of Cleanroom Standards

It is best to start this section of the book by giving some indication of the size of particles used in cleanroom standards. The unit of measurement is a micrometre, one micrometre (1 μm) being one millionth of a metre. Figure 3.1 shows a drawing comparing particle sizes. A human hair, a size that can be readily appreciated, is approximately 70–100 μm in diameter. Another size that helps to put particle sizes into perspective is the size of particle that can be seen on a surface. This is approximately 50 μm in diameter, although this varies quite considerably depending on the acuteness of sight of the person, the colour of the particle and the colour of the background.

Cleanrooms are classified by the cleanliness of their air. The most easily understood classification of cleanrooms is the one used in the earlier versions (A to D) of Federal Standard 209 of the USA. This classification has been superseded by the last version of the Federal Standard (E) and now by the International Standard ISO 14644-1. However, this old classification is still widely used. In the older Federal Standards (A to D), the number of particles equal to, and greater than, 0.5 μm were measured in one cubic foot of air and this count used to classify a room. The most recent Federal Standard 209 (E version) accepted a metric nomenclature, but in 1999, ISO 14644-1 was published. This standard has been adopted by all countries in the European Union and is now being adopted by other countries.

In this book, cleanroom classifications are given according to ISO 14644-1, with the Federal Standard 209 classification given in parentheses, e.g. ISO Class 5 (Class 100).

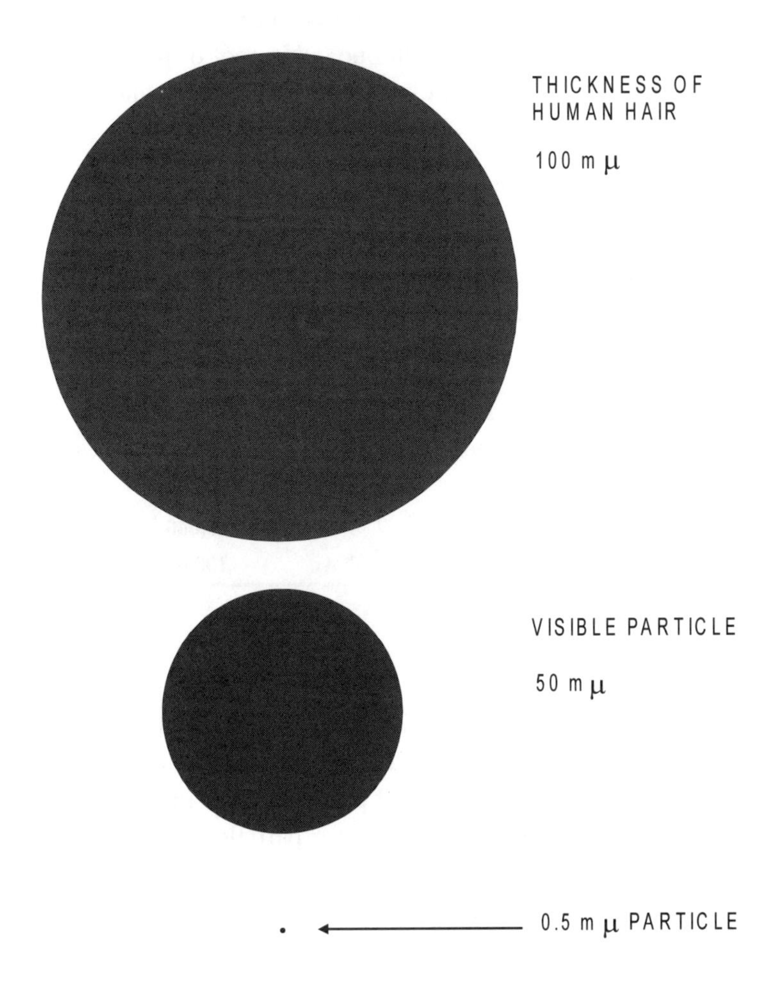

Figure 3.1 Comparison of particle diameters

3.3 Federal Standard 209

3.3.1 The earlier Federal Standards 209 (A to D)

The first Federal Standard 209 was published in 1963 in the USA and titled "Cleanroom and Work Station Requirements, Controlled Environments". It was revised in 1966 (209A), 1973 (B), 1987 (C), 1988 (D) and 1992 (E). The cleanroom class limits, given in the earlier 209 A to D versions, are shown in Table 3.1. The actual class of a cleanroom is found by measuring the number of particles ≥ 0.5 μm in one cubic foot of room air, and determining which class limit is not exceeded; this is the cleanroom classification.

Table 3.1 Federal Standard 209 D class limits

Class		**Particles**	**/ ft^3**		
	≥ 0.1 μm	≥ 0.2 μm	≥ 0.3 μm	**≥ 0.5 μm**	≥ 5.0 μm
1	35	7.5	3	**1**	NA
10	350	75	30	**10**	NA
100	NA	750	300	**100**	NA
1,000	NA	NA	NA	**1,000**	7
10,000	NA	NA	NA	**10,000**	70
100,000	NA	NA	NA	**100,000**	700

3.3.2 Federal Standard 209 E

In Federal Standard 209 E the airborne concentrations in the room are given in metric units, i.e. per m^3 and the classifications defined as the logarithm of the airborne concentration of particles ≥ 0.5 μm per m^3. For example, a Class M3 room has a class limit for particles ≥ 0.5 μm of $1000/m^3$. The logarithm of 1000 is 3, which is the class. This is shown in Table 3.2. The current version is available from the Institute of Environmental Sciences and Technology in the USA. Their contact information is given in Chapter 4.

Table 3.2 Federal Standard 209 E class limits

Class Name		**Class Limits**									
		≥ 0.1µm		≥ 0.2µm		≥ 0.3µm		≥ 0.5µm		≥ 5µm	
		Volume Units		Volume Units		Volume Units		Volume Units		Volume Units	
SI	English	(m^3)	(ft^3)	(m^3)	(ft^3)	(m^3)	(ft^3)	(m^3)	(ft^3)	(m^3)	(ft^3)
M 1		350	9.91	75.7	2.14	30.9	0.875	10.0	0.283	--	--
M 1.5	1	1 240	35.0	265	7.50	106	3.00	35.3	1.00	--	--
M 2		3 500	99.1	757	21.4	309	8.75	100	2.83	--	--
M 2.5	10	12 400	350	2 650	75.0	1 060	30.0	353	10.0	--	--
M 3		35 000	991	7 570	214	3 090	87.5	1 000	28.3	--	--
M 3.5	100	--	--	26 500	750	10 600	300	3 530	100	--	--
M 4		--	--	75 700	2 140	30 900	875	10 000	283	--	--
M 4.5	1 000	--	--	--	--	--	--	35 300	1 000	247	7.00
M 5		--	--	--	--	--	--	100 000	2 830	618	17.5
M 5.5	10 000	--	--	--	--	--	--	353 000	10 000	2 470	70.0
M 6		--	--	--	--	--	--	1 000 000	28 300	6 180	175
M 6.5	100 000	--	--	--	--	--	--	3 350 000	100 000	24 700	700
M 7		--	--	--	--	--	--	10 000 000	283 000	61 800	1 750

3.4 ISO Standard 14644-1

The International Organization for Standards (ISO) is developing a series of cleanroom standards. These cover a wide variety of important cleanroom issues such as design, testing, operation and biocontamination. The first document, published in 1999, is ISO 14644-1 and entitled 'Classification of Air Cleanliness'. This gives the cleanroom classification method. Other standards are also available and these are discussed in the Chapter 4. Information on where to purchase the ISO 14644-1 standard is also given in the Chapter 4.

The ISO classification is based on the following equation:

$$Cn = 10^{N} \times \left[\frac{0.1}{D}\right]^{2.08} \tag{3.1}$$

where:

Cn is the maximum permitted concentration (in particles/m^3 of air) of airborne particles that are equal to, or larger, than the considered particle size.

Cn is rounded to the nearest whole number, using no more than three significant figures.

N is the ISO classification number, which shall not exceed the value of 9. Intermediate ISO classification numbers may be specified, with 0.1 the smallest permitted increment of N.

D is the considered particle size in μm.

0.1 is a constant with a dimension of μm.

From equation 3.1, the maximum permitted airborne concentration of particles, i.e. the class limit can be calculated for any given particle size. Shown in Table 3.3 are the classes selected by ISO 14644-1 to illustrate class limits.

It should be noted that there is a crossover to the Federal Standard 209 classes. If the particle concentration/m^3 in the ISO standard is divided by 35.2 the count is converted to counts/ft^3 . The equivalent Federal Standard

209 classification is then found in Table 3.3 at the 0.5 μm size, e.g. an ISO Class 5 is equivalent to Federal Standard 209 Class 100 or M3.5.

Table 3.3 Selected ISO 14644-1 airborne particulate cleanliness classes for cleanrooms and clean zones

ISO Classification number	Maximum concentration limits (particles/m^3 of air) for particles equal to and larger than the considered sizes shown below					
	≥0.1μm	≥0.2μm	≥0.3μm	≥0.5μm	≥1μm	≥5.0μm
ISO Class 1	10	2				
ISO Class 2	100	24	10	4		
ISO Class 3	1 000	237	102	35	8	
ISO Class 4	10 000	2 370	1 020	352	83	
ISO Class 5	100 000	23 700	10 200	3 520	832	29
ISO Class 6	1 000 000	237 000	102 000	35 200	8 320	293
ISO Class 7				352 000	83 200	2 930
ISO Class 8				3 520 000	832 000	29 300
ISO Class 9				35 200 000	8 320 000	293 000

Table 3.4 Comparison between selected equivalent classes of FS 209 and ISO 14644-1

ISO 14644-1 Classes	Class 3	Class 4	Class 5	Class6	Class 7	Class 8
FS 209 Classes	Class 1	Class 10	Class 100	Class 1000	Class 10 000	Class 6 100 000

Given in ISO 14644-1 is the same information in a graphical form. This is shown in Figure 3.2. It should be appreciated that the airborne particle concentration of a given cleanroom is dependent on the particle generating activities going on in the room.

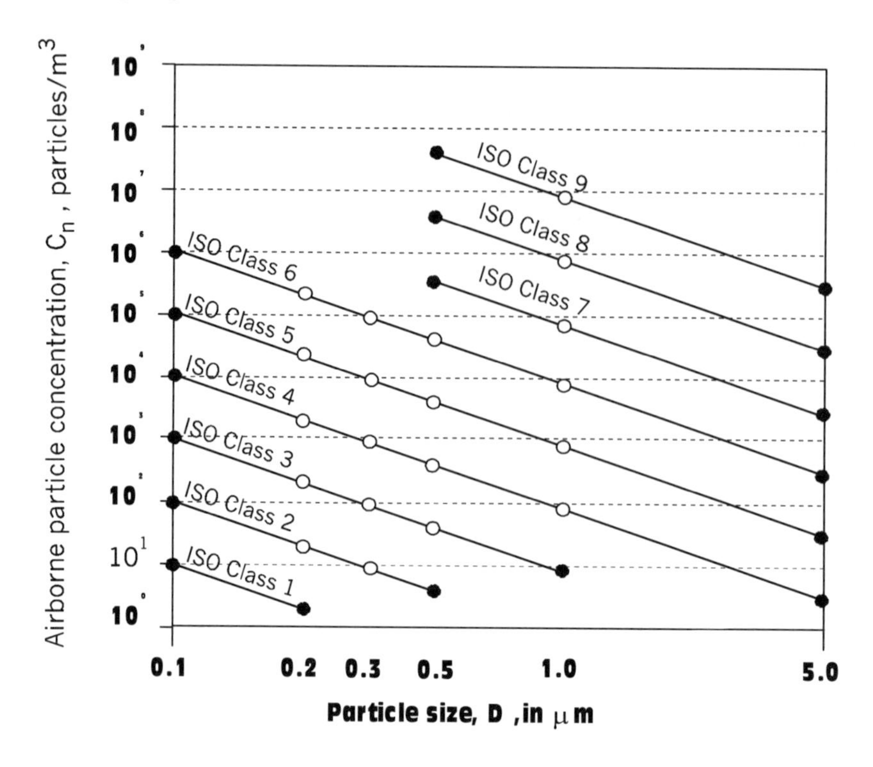

Figure 3.2 Graphical representation of ISO-class concentration limits for selected ISO classes.

If a room is empty, a very low particle concentration can be achieved, this closely reflecting the quality of air supplied. If the room has production equipment in it that is operating, there should be a greater particle concentration, but the greatest concentration occurs when the room is in full production. The classification of the room may therefore be carried out in these different occupancy states.

The occupancy states defined in ISO 14644-1 are as follows:

As built: the condition where the installation is complete with all services connected and functioning, but with no production equipment, materials or personnel present.
At-rest: The condition where the installation is complete with equipment installed and operating in a manner agreed between the customer and supplier, but with no personnel present.
Operational: The condition where the installation is functioning in the specified manner, with the specified number of personnel present and working in the manner agreed upon.

The ISO 14644-1 standard also gives a method by which the standard of a cleanroom may be ascertained by measuring particles at various sampling locations. The method for determining the number of sampling locations, the sampling volume and counting the number of airborne particles is similar to Federal Standard 209 E and discussed in Chapter 13 of this book.

ISO 14644-1 also includes a method for specifying a cleanroom using particles outside the size range given in Table 3.2. Smaller particles known in the standard as 'ultrafine' (≤ 0.1 μm) are of particular importance in the semiconductor industry and the large 'macroparticles' (≥ 5 μm) are of use in industries, such as parts of the medical device industry, where small particles are of no practical importance. Fibres can also be specified. The M descriptor method employed with macroparticles uses the format:

'M(a; b);c'

where

a is the maximum permitted concentration/m^3
b is the equivalent diameter.
c is the specified measurement method.

An example would be: 'M(1 000; 10 μm to 20 μm); cascade impactor followed by microscopic sizing and counting'. A similar classification method is used with 'ultrafine' particles.

3.5 Pharmaceutical Cleanroom Classification

Cleanrooms used for pharmaceutical manufacturing have their own standards. The two most widely used are those published by the European Union and the USA.

3.5.1 European Union Guide to Good Manufacturing Practice

The most recent pharmaceutical standard used in Europe came into operation on January 1997. This is called 'The rules governing medicinal products in the European Union. Volume 4. Good manufacturing practices - Medicinal products for human and veterinary use'. It is often called the European Union Guide to Good Manufacturing Products (EU GGMP). This is available in various languages of the EU. Information as to where the standard can be obtained is given in Chapter 4.

For the manufacture of sterile medicinal products four grades of airborne cleanliness are given. The airborne particulate classification for these grades is given in Table 3.4.

Table 3.4 Airborne classification in the EU GGMP

	Maximum permitted number of particles/m^3 equal to or above			
Grade	**at rest (b)**		**in operation**	
	0.5 μm	5 μm	0.5 μm	5 μm
A	3 500	0	3 500	0
B(a)	3 500	0	350 000	2 000
C(a)	350 000	2 000	3 500 000	20 000
D(a)	3 500 000	20 000	not defined (c)	not defined (c)

Notes
(a) In order to reach the B, C and D air grades, the number of air changes should be related to the size of the room and the equipment and personnel present in the room. The air system should be provided with appropriate filters such as HEPA for grades A, B and C.
(b) The guidance given for the maximum permitted number of particles in the 'at rest' condition corresponds approximately to the US Federal Standard 209 E and the ISO classifications as follows: grades A and B correspond with class 100, M 3.5, ISO 5; grade C with class 10 000, M 5.5, ISO 7 and grade D with class 100 000, M 6.5, ISO 8.
(c) The requirement and limit for this area will depend on the nature of the operations carried out.

The particulate conditions given Table 3.4 for the 'at rest' state should be achieved after a short 'clean up' period of 15–20 minutes (guidance value), after the completion of operations.

Examples of operations to be carried out in the various grades are given in the Table 3.5. The particulate conditions for a grade A zone that is in operation should be maintained in the zone immediately surrounding the product whenever the product or open container is exposed to the environment. It is accepted that it may not always be possible to demonstrate conformity with particulate standards at the point of fill when filling is in progress, due to the generation of particles or droplets from the product itself.

Table 3.5 Examples of cleanroom conditions required for different operations

Grade	Examples of Operations for Terminally Sterilised Products
A	Filling of products, when unusually at risk
C	Preparation of solutions, when unusually at risk. Filling of products
D	Preparation of solutions and components for subsequent filling
Grade	**Examples of Operations for Aseptic Preparations**
A	Aseptic preparation and filling
C	Preparation of solutions to be filtered
D	Handling of components after washing.

Microbiological monitoring is also required to demonstrate the microbiological cleanliness of the cleanroom during production. The recommended limits are given in Table 3.6.

Table 3.6 Recommended limits for microbial contamination

Grade	**Air Sample** cfu/m^3	**Settle Plates** (diam. 90 mm), cfu/4 hours (b)	**Contact Plates** (diam. 55 mm), cfu/plate	**Glove Print** 5 fingers cfu/glove
A	< 1	< 1	< 1	< 1
B	10	5	5	5
C	100	50	25	-
D	200	100	50	-

Notes

(a) These are average values.
(b) Individual settle plates may be exposed for less than 4 hours.
(c) Appropriate alert and action limits should be set for the results of particulate and microbiological monitoring. If these limits are exceeded, operating procedures should prescribe corrective action.

The air classification required for a cleanroom that has an isolator used to protect against contamination depends on the design of the isolator and its application. It should be controlled and for aseptic processing be at least grade D.

Blow/fill/seal equipment used for aseptic production, which is fitted with an effective grade A air shower, may be installed in at least a grade C environment, provided that grade A/B clothing is used. The environment should comply with the viable and non-viable limits 'at rest', and the viable limit only when in 'operation'. Blow/fill/seal equipment used for the production of products for terminal sterilisation should be installed in at least a grade D environment.

3.5.2 *Guideline on Sterile Drug Products Produced by Aseptic Processing.*

This document is produced by the Food and Drug Administration (FDA) in the USA and published in 1987. Information on how to obtain this document can be found in the Chapter 4.

The FDA defines two areas in aseptic processing that are of particular importance to drug product quality. These are the 'critical area' and the 'controlled area'. A 'critical area' is described in the FDA document as:

> *'one in which the sterilized dosage form, containers, and closures are exposed to the environment. Activities that are conducted in this area include manipulations of these sterilized materials/product prior to and during filling/closing operations'.*

The 'controlled area' is described as:

> *'an area in which it is important to control the environment, is the area where unsterilized product, in-process materials, and container/closures are prepared. This includes areas where components are compounded, and where components, in-process materials, drug products and drug product contact surfaces of equipment, containers, and closures, after final rinse of such surfaces, are exposed to the plant environment'.*

The environmental requirements for these two areas given in the Guide are as follows:

3.5.2.1 Critical areas

The FDA guidelines give the following information:

> *'Air in the immediate proximity of exposed sterilized containers/closures and filling/closing operations is of acceptable particulate quality when it has a per-cubic-foot particle count of no more than 100 in a size range of 0.5 micron and larger (Class 100) when measured not more than one foot away from the work site, and upstream of the air flow, during filling/closing operations. The agency recognizes that some powder filling operations may generate high levels of powder particulates which, by their nature, do not*

pose a risk of product contamination. It may not, in these cases, be feasible to measure air quality within the one foot distance and still differentiate "background noise" levels of powder particles from air contaminants which can impeach product quality. In these instances, it is nonetheless important to sample the air in a manner, which to the extent possible characterises the true level of extrinsic particulate contamination to which the product is exposed.

Air in critical areas should be supplied at the point of use as HEPA filtered laminar flow air, having a velocity sufficient to sweep particulate matter away from the filling/closing area. Normally, a velocity of 90 feet per minute, plus or minus 20%, is adequate, although higher velocities may be needed where the operations generate high levels of particulates or where equipment configuration disrupts laminar flow.

Air should also be of a high microbial quality. An incidence of no more than one colony forming unit per 10 cubic feet is considered as attainable and desirable.

Critical areas should have a positive pressure differential relative to adjacent less clean areas; a pressure differential of 0.05 inch of water is acceptable'.

3.5.2.2 Controlled areas

The FDA Guidelines give the following information:

'Air in controlled areas is generally of acceptable particulate quality if it has a per-cubic-foot particle count of not more than 100,000 in a size range of 0.5 micron and larger (Class 100,000) when measured in the vicinity of the exposed articles during periods of activity. With regard to microbial quality, an incidence of no more than 25 colony forming units per 10 cubic feet is acceptable.

In order to maintain air quality in controlled areas, it is important to achieve a sufficient air flow and a positive pressure differential relative to adjacent uncontrolled areas. In this regard, an air flow sufficient to achieve at least 20 air changes per hour and, in general, a pressure differential of at least 0.05 inch of water (with all doors closed), are acceptable. When doors are open, outward airflow should be sufficient to minimize ingress of contamination'.

Acknowledgements

Table 3.3 and Figure 3.2, as well as extracts of ISO 14644-1 are reproduced by permission of the British Standards Institution.

4

Information Sources

It is important to be able to obtain current information about cleanrooms through the latest standards, books, recommended practices, magazines and other documents, as well as through the Internet. This chapter gives such information. This information was current when this book was published but communication details are continually changing. It is hoped that this chapter can be updated from time-to-time but readers should be aware of the possibility that the information may not be current.

4.1 The International Confederation of Contamination Control Societies (ICCCS)

The ICCCS is a confederation of societies that have an interest in cleanroom technology. The present membership is as follows:

ACCS: Australian Contamination Control Society, Australia
ASCCA: Associazione per lo Studio ed il Controllo della Contaminazione Ambientale, Italy
ASENMCO: Association of Engineers for Microcontamination Control, Russia
ASPEC: Association pour la Prevention et l'Etude de la Contamination, France
BCW: Belgian Cleanroom Workclub, A.S.B.L., Belgium
CCCS: Chinese Contamination Control Society, China
GAA-RR of DIN/VDI: Gemeinschaftsarbeitsausschuß Reinraumtechnik, GAA-RR, within DIN and VDI, Germany
ICS: Irish Cleanroom Society, Ireland

IEST: Institute of Environmental Sciences and Technology, USA
JACA: Japanese Air Cleaning Association, Japan
R^3 Nordic: Renhetsteknik och Rena Rum, Denmark, Finland, Norway and Sweden
KACRA: Republic of Korea, South Korea
SBCC: Sociedade Brasileira de Controle de Contaminacáo, Brazil
SEE: Society of Environmental Engineers, UK
SRRT: Schweizerische Gesellschaft für Reinraumtechnik, Switzerland
S2C2: Scottish Society for Contamination Control, Scotland;
VCCN: Vereniging Contamination Control Nederland, the Netherlands.

Anyone who is interested in the design, testing or operation of cleanrooms is advised to join their local society to keep their cleanroom knowledge up-to-date. A current list of the secretariates of member societies and their contact information is available on the ICCCS web site (www.icccs.org) or through its Secretariate at the following address:

ICCCS Secretariate
Postbus 311
3830 A J Leusden
The Netherlands.
Tel: +31 33 43 45 752
Fax: + 31 33 43 21 581
E-mail: icccs @ tvvl.nl

4.2 International Cleanroom Standards

4.2.1 ISO standards

A range of cleanroom standards is being produced by the International Organization for Standardization (ISO). Various committees of experts, nominated by countries throughout the world, are writing these standards.

The standards that have been published, or being written at the time of publication of this book, are as follows:

4.2.1.1 ISO 14644

This consists of the following parts, under the general title 'Cleanrooms and Associated Controlled Environments':

Part 1: Classification of air cleanliness
This gives the airborne particle limits for different standards of cleanrooms. It also gives the methods that should be used to measure the airborne particles when testing a cleanroom to determine its class.
Part 2: Specifications for testing and monitoring to prove continued compliance with ISO14644-1
This gives information, including time intervals, for testing a cleanroom to show that it still complies with the ISO 14644-1 standard.
Part 3: Metrology and test methods
This gives a description of the test methods that should be used to test the cleanroom to show that it is working correctly.
Part 4: Design, construction, and startup
This gives general guidance as to how a cleanroom should be designed, constructed and made ready for handing over to the user.
Part 5 Operation
This gives general advice on how to run a cleanroom.
Part 6: Terms and definitions
This is a collection of all the definitions of terms used in the ISO cleanroom standards.
Part 7: Separative enclosures (clean air hoods, gloveboxes, isolator, mini environments)
This gives information on clean air devices such as isolators and minienvironments.
Part 8: Molecular contamination
This gives information on gaseous contamination in cleanrooms.

4.2.1.2 ISO 14698

This consists of the following parts under the general title 'Cleanrooms and Associated Controlled Environments–Biocontamination Control':

Part 1: General principles and methods
This gives information on how to establish methods for measuring micro-organisms in the cleanroom.
Part 2: Evaluation and interpretation of biocontamination data
This gives information on how to deal with the results obtained from measuring micro-organisms in a cleanroom.

These standards are also available throughout the world from the various national standard organisations; they are also available in some national languages. For further information on the various ISO members world-wide, where standards can be bought, you should visit the Internet at www.iso.ch/addre.html or contact:

International Organization for Standardization (ISO)
1 rue de Varembe
Case postale 56
CH-1211 Geneve 20
Switzerland.
Tel: +41 22 749 0111
Fax: +41 22 733 3430
Web site: www.iso.ch

Information about the availability of these standards is available in the UK from the British Standards Institution using the following contact information:

British Standards Institution
Customer Services
389 Chiswick High Road
London W4 4AL
UK.
Tel +44 (0)20 8996 9001
Fax +44(0)20 8996 7001
Web site: www.bsi-global.com

In the USA these standards are available from the Institute of Environmental Sciences and Technology (IEST) using the following communication details:

Institute of Environmental Sciences and Technology
940 East Northwest Highway
Mount Prospect
Illinois, 60056,
USA.
Tel: +1 708 255 1561
Fax: +1 708 255 1699
Web site: www iest.org

4.2.2 Federal Standard 209 E

Although this standard is being superseded by ISO 14644-1, it is still in use throughout the world. It is available from IEST, their communication details being given immediately above (Section 4.2.1.2).

4.2.3 Pharmaceutical standards

The two most commonly used standards concerned with pharmaceutical cleanrooms are available from the European Union and the Federal Drug Association (FDA) in the USA.

4.2.3.1. The European Union Guide to Good Manufacturing Practice (EU GGMP)

This can be downloaded free from the Internet at the following address: http://pharmacos.eudra.org. It is contained in the 'units activities' section under the heading 'Eudralex'. Volume 4 is the correct document.

This document is also available in various languages of the countries within the EU and obtained from bookshops in these countries. Information as to where these outlets are to be found can be obtained from:

Office for Official Publications of the European Communities
2 rue Mercier
L-2985 Luxembourg.
Tel +352 29 29-42455 Fax: +352 29 29-42758
Web site: http://eur-op.eu.int

The above office encourages customers to purchase from their local distributors, contact information being published in the Internet site. In the UK, the EU GGMP is available from:
Stationery Office
PO Box 29
Norwich, NR3 1GN
UK.
Tel: +44 (0) 870 600 5522
Fax: +44 (0) 870 600 5533
Web site: www.the-stationery-office.co.uk

4.2.3.2 Guideline on Sterile Drug Products Produced by Aseptic Processing

This can be downloaded free from the web site of the FDA Centre for Drug Evaluation and Research at: www.fda.gov. After opening the FDA site you should click on 'Drugs'. The document is available, at the time of writing, in their 'Regulatory Guidance' section where it may be found in the 'Guidance Documents Web Page' under the 'Compliance' heading. It is also possible (but not encouraged) to get it from the following address:

FDA Drug Information Branch
HFD-210
5600 Fishers Lane
Rockville
MD 20857
USA.
Tel: +1-301-827-4527
Web site: www.fda.gov

4.3 Cleanroom Books

The following is a list of books (in alphabetical order) written in the English language that I know to be available through a bookstore. I would be pleased to receive any other titles so that the list can be extended.

1. ***Cleanroom Design*** edited by Whyte, W. (1991). Wiley, Chichester, UK. ISBN 0-471-92814-3.
2. ***Clean Room Design*** by Ljungvist, B. and Reinmuller, B. (1997). Interpharm Press, Buffalo Grove, IL 60089, USA.
3. ***Cleanrooms-Facilities and Practices*** by Kozicki, M. N. with Hoenig, S. A. and Robinson, P. A. (1991). Van Nostrand Reinhold, New York. ISBN 0-442-31950-9.
4. ***Contamination Control and Cleanrooms*** by Lieberman, A. (1992). Van Nostrand Reinhold, New York. ISBN 0-442-00574-1.
5. ***Handbook of Contamination Control in Microelectronics*** Edited by Toliver, D. L. (1988). Noyes Publications, Park Ridge, NJ, USA.
6. ***Introduction to Contamination Control and Cleanroom Technology*** by Ramstorp, M. (2000). Wiley-VCH. ISBN 3-527-30142-9.
7. ***Isolator Technology*** by Wagner, C. M. and Akers, J.E. (1995). Interpharm Press, Buffalo Grove, IL 60089, USA.
8. ***Isolator Technology – a Practical Guide*** by Coles, T (1998). Interpharm Press, Buffalo Grove, IL 60089, USA.
9. ***Practical Cleanroom Design*** by Schneider, R K. (1995). Business News Publishing Company, Troy, MI, USA. ISBN 1-885863-03-9.

4.4 Recommended Practices and Guides of the Institute of Environmental Sciences and Technology (IEST)

The IEST in the USA produce a large number of Recommended Practices (RPs) and Guides that cover many topics. They are an invaluable source of information and are available from:

Institute of Environmental Sciences and Technology
940 East Northwest Highway
Mount Prospect
Illinois, 60056, USA.
Tel: +1 708 255 1561
Fax: +1 708 255 1699
Web site: www.iest.org

4.4.1 IEST Recommended Practices (RPs)

The following RPs are available:

IEST-RP-CC001: HEPA and ULPA filters
This covers the basic provisions for HEPA and ULPA filter units. Six levels of performance and six grades of construction are included.
IEST-RP-CC002: Laminar flow clean-air devices
Covers definitions, procedures for evaluating performance, and major requirements of unidirectional flow clean air devices
IEST-RP-CC003: Garments required in cleanrooms and controlled environments
Provides guidance for the specification, testing, selection and maintenance of garments use in cleanrooms.
IEST-RP-CC004: Evaluating wiping materials used in cleanrooms and other controlled environments
Describes methods for testing wipers used in cleanrooms for characteristics related to cleanliness and function.
IEST-RP-CC005: Cleanroom gloves and finger cots
Describes parameters and tests that apply to gloves and finger cots.
IEST-RP-CC006: Testing cleanrooms
Describes tests to evaluate and characterise the overall performance of the cleanroom and clean zone system.
IEST-RP-CC007: Testing ULPA filters
Describes a test procedure for production testing of ULPA filters for particle penetration and pressure drop.

IEST-RP-CC008: Gas-phase adsorber cells
Covers the design and testing of modular gas-phase adsorber cells for use where high efficiency removal of gaseous contaminants is required.
IEST-RD-CC009: Compendium of standards, practices, methods, and similar documents relating to contamination control
Lists standards, practices, methods, technical orders, specifications, and similar documents developed by government, industry and technical societies in the United States and other countries.
IEST-RD-CC011: A glossary of terms and definitions relating to contamination control
Defines terms relating to contamination control and contains lists of frequently used abbreviations and acronyms.
IEST-RP-CC012: Considerations in cleanroom design
Makes recommendations regarding factors to consider in the design of cleanroom facilities.
IEST-RP-CC013: Equipment calibration or validation procedures
Covers definitions and procedures for calibrating instruments used for testing clean rooms and intervals of calibration.
IEST-RP-CC015: Cleanroom production and support equipment
Suggests approaches for the design, installation and operation of production and support equipment used within a cleanroom to minimise the contribution of that equipment to the contamination of the product.
IEST-RP-CC016: The rate of deposition of nonvolatile residue in cleanrooms
Provides a method for determining the rate of deposition of nonvolatile residue (NVR) on surfaces in cleanrooms.
IEST-RP-CC018: Cleanroom housekeeping-operating and monitoring procedures
Provides guidance for establishing housekeeping procedures and monitoring surface cleanliness.
IEST-RP-CC020: Substrates and forms for documentation in cleanrooms
Provides guidance for substrates and forms used in cleanrooms for the purpose of documentation.

IEST-RP-CC021: Testing HEPA and ULPA filter media
Discusses test methods for physical and filtration properties of high efficiency particulate air and ultra low penetration air filtration media.
IEST-RP-CC022: Electrostatic charge in cleanrooms and other controlled environments
Discusses methods for specifying and evaluating the effectiveness of techniques for controlling electrostatic charge.
IEST-RP-CC023: Microorganisms in cleanrooms
Provides guidelines for the control and quantitative measurement of viable air and surface contamination.
IEST-RP-CC024: Measuring and reporting vibration in microelectronic facilities
Discusses equipment used in the manufacture, measurement and inspection of integrated circuits sensitive to vibration and sound in the microelectronics industry.
IEST-RP-CC026: Cleanroom operations
Provides guidance for maintaining the integrity of the cleanroom during preparation of supplies and materials, modification of the facility, and installation and repair of equipment.
IEST-RP-CC027: Personnel practices and procedures in cleanroom and controlled environments
Provides a basis for establishing personnel procedures and the development of training programs for cleanrooms.
IEST-RP-CC029: Automotive paint spray applications
Provides recommended procedures for controlling dirt in paint spray operations
IEST-RD-CC031: Building code reference handbook: a guide to alternative code compliance issues in the semiconductor industry
This document is a reference guide for code issues that require alternative compliance to design, construct or operation of semiconductor facilities.
IEST-RP-CC034: HEPA and ULPA filter leak tests
Covers definitions, equipment and procedures for leak testing filters in the factory and in the cleanroom.

4.4.2 IEST Guides

The following Guides are available to complement ISO 14644-1 and ISO 14644-2:

IEST-G-CC1001: Counting airborne particles for classification and monitoring of cleanrooms and clean zones
This guide provides information on methods used to sample air in clean environments using a discrete particle counter to determine concentrations of airborne particles.
IEST-G-CC1002: Determination of the concentration of airborne ultrafine particles.
This supplements the coverage of procedures for determining the concentration of ultrafine particles as provided by ISO 14644-1.
IEST-G-CC1003: Measurement of airborne macroparticles.
This covers the sampling of macroparticles, these being the larger particles to be found in cleanrooms.
IEST-G-CC1004: Sequential-sampling plan for use in classification of the particle cleanliness of air in cleanrooms and clean zones. This expands the coverage of sequential sampling as introduced in ISO 14644-1.

4.5 Cleanroom Journals and Magazines

4.5.1 Free distribution

The following magazines are often distributed free of charge. However, this free circulation may be restricted to the country of publication, and to individuals that the magazine publishing companies consider to have *bona fide* cleanroom credentials.
A2C2–Journal of Advancing Applications in Contamination Control
This publication is published monthly by:

A2C2
Vicon Publishing, Inc.
62 Route 101A

Ste. 3
Amherst, NH 03031
USA.
Telephone +1-603-672-9997
Fax: +1-603-672-3028
Web site: www.a2c2.com

CleanRooms
Cleanrooms is monthly magazine produced by:

CleanRooms
98 Spit Brook Road
Fifth Floor
Nashua NH 03062
USA.
Tel: +1 603 891 0123
Fax: +1 603 891 9200
Web site: www.cleanrooms.com

Cleanroom Technology
This publication is published monthly by:

Polygon Media Ltd
Tubshill House
London Road
Sevenoaks
Kent, TN13 1BY, UK.
Tel: +44 (0)1732 470000
Fax: +44 (0)1732 470047
Web site: www.cleanroom-technology.eu.com

Micro Magazine
This publication is concerned with defect reduction and yield enhancement strategies for semiconductor and advance microelectronics and is published monthly by:

Canon Communications
11444 W. Olympic Blvd
Ste. 900
Los Angeles
CA 90064
USA
Telephone (for subscriptions) +1-651 686 7824
Fax (for subscriptions): +1-651 686 4883
Web site: www.micromagazine.com

4.5.2 Journals and magazines available on subscription.

Journal of the Institute of Environmental Sciences and Technology

This is available free to the members of IEST, or by subscription. It covers a wider field of interest than cleanrooms, but usually has at least one article about cleanroom related issues in each issue. It is available from:

Institute of Environmental Sciences and Technology
940 East Northwest Highway
Mount Prospect
Illinois, 60056
USA.
Tel: +1 847 255 1561
Fax: +1 847 255 1699
Web site: www.iest.org

European Journal of Parenteral Sciences

This is a quarterly journal published by the Parenteral Society in the UK and is the official journal of the European Sterile Products Confederation (ESPC). It usually has articles concerned with contamination control in pharmaceutical manufacturing. Available from:

European Journal of Parenteral Sciences
Euromed Communications Ltd

The Old Surgery
Liphook Road,
Hastlemere
Surrey
England, GU27 1NL, UK
Tel: +44-(0)1428 656665
Fax: +44 (0)1428 656643
Web site: www.euromed.uk.com/ejps

PDA Journal of Parenteral Science
The Parenteral Drug Association (PDA) in the USA publishes this journal. It usually has articles concerned with contamination control in pharmaceutical manufacturing. It is available from:

Parenteral Drug Association
7500 Old Georgetown Road
Suite 620
Bethesda, MD 20814
USA.
Tel: +1 301 986 0293
Fax: +1 301 986 0296
Web site:www.pda.org

4.6 Sources of Pharmaceutical Cleanroom Documents

Interpharm Catalog
A catalogue of technical books, regulatory documents, productivity software and audio-visual training tools is available from:

Interpharm Press
15 Inverness Way East
Englewood
CO 80112-9240
USA.

Tel: +1 303 662 9101
Fax: +1 303 754 3953
Website: www.interpharm.com

Parenteral Society
This Society has a selection of books, monographs and videos. They can be reached at:

Parenteral Society
99 Ermin Street
Stratton St Margaret
Swindon
Wilts, SN3 4Nl, UK.
Tel: +44 (0)1793 824254
Fax: +44 (0) 1793 832551
Web site: www.parenteral.org.uk

Parenteral Drug Association. This society has a selection of books, monographs and videos. They can be reached at:

Parenteral Drug Association
7500 Old Georgetown Road
Suite 620
Bethesda, MD 20814, USA.
Tel +1 301 986 0293
Fax +1 301 986 0296
Web site: www.pda.org

4.7 International Cleanroom Forum

This is a questions and answer forum on the Internet. It is sponsored by the International Confederation of Contamination Control Societies (ICCCS) and maintained by the Scottish Society for Contamination Control (S2C2).

Experts are available to answer simple or complex questions about cleanrooms. It can be accessed at either www. s2c2.co.uk or www.icccs.org.

5

The Design of Turbulently Ventilated and Ancillary Cleanrooms

5.1 Turbulently Ventilated Cleanrooms

The ventilation principles of turbulently ventilated cleanrooms are similar to those found in most air conditioned rooms, such as offices and shops. The air is supplied by an air conditioning plant through diffusers in the ceiling. Figure 5.1 is a diagram of a simple turbulently ventilated cleanroom.

This type of cleanroom is called a 'turbulently ventilated' cleanroom in this book as the air moves in a turbulent-random way within the room. This distinguishes it from a unidirectional flow cleanroom, where the air enters through filters across the whole ceiling, or wall, and flows in a unidirectional manner across the cleanroom. A turbulently ventilated room is also known as a 'non unidirectional' cleanroom; however, this does not describe the airflow as well.

The design of a turbulently ventilated cleanroom differs from an ordinary air conditioned room in a number of ways. These are:

- The air supply volume is much greater.
- High efficiency air filters are used and normally fitted where the air enters the cleanroom.

- The air movement within the cleanroom assists in the removal of contamination.
- The room is pressurised so that air flows out to less-clean adjacent areas.
- Construction material and finishes are of a high standard.

These attributes of a turbulently ventilated cleanroom are now discussed in more detail.

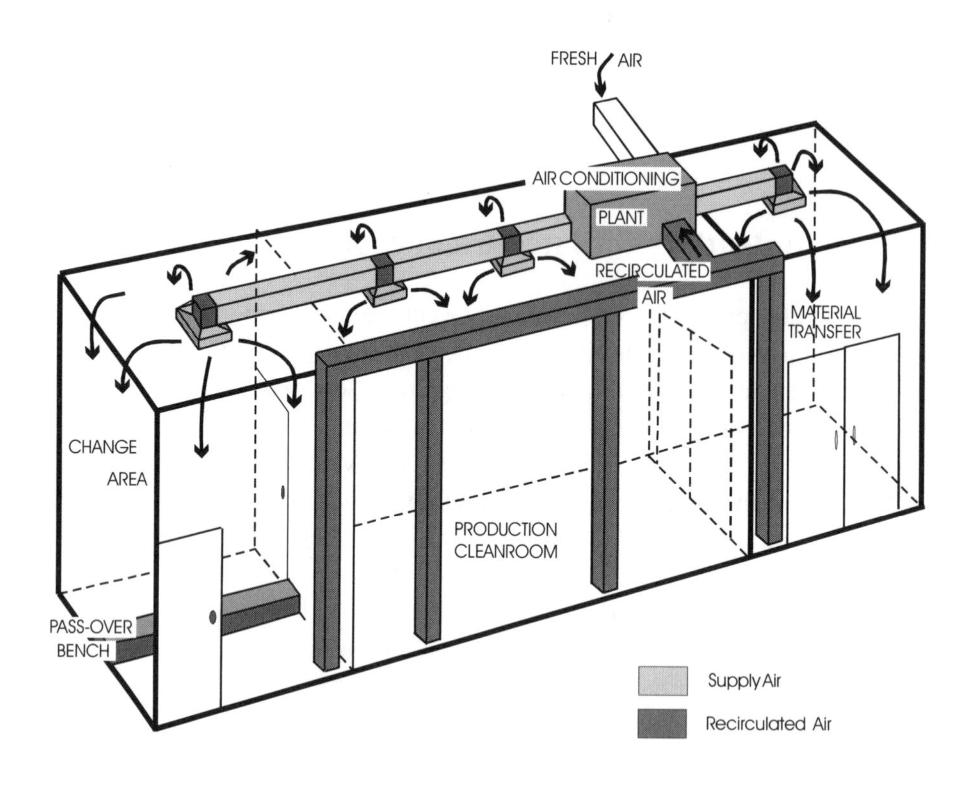

Figure 5.1 A turbulently ventilated cleanroom

5.1.1 Air supply

A normal air conditioned room, such as an office or shop, will be supplied with just sufficient air to achieve comfort conditions; this may be in the region of 2 – 10 air changes per hour. However, a typical turbulently ventilated cleanroom is likely to have between 10 and 100 air changes per hour. This additional air is required to dilute the contamination dispersed into the room and to reduce it to a concentration specified in a cleanroom standard.

Cleanrooms require large quantities of air that is air conditioned and filtered to an very high standard. To ensure an economic design, it is essential that the cleanroom air is recirculated back through the air conditioning plant. However, it is also necessary to provide fresh outside air for the health of personnel working in the cleanroom and to pressurise the cleanroom against outside contamination. Normally between 2% and 10% of the total air supply is fresh air; large airtight rooms require a lower percentage than small less-airtight rooms. If air extract systems are used to remove contamination from around machinery or processes, then the percentage of fresh air will have to be increased to compensate.

When designing a ventilation system for a room like an office, it is necessary to calculate the amount of air required to keep the room cool; this is dependent on the heat generated in the room. In cleanrooms it is quite common to find that production equipment produces large quantities of heat. It is therefore not unusual to find that the amount of air required to cool the room is similar to that required to achieve the correct clean air standard.

Air changes per hour are a common way of expressing air dilution in the room and give an indication of the cleanliness of a room. However, the airborne cleanliness of a turbulently ventilated cleanroom is really dependent on the volume of air supplied to the room in a given time. The airborne cleanliness is also related to the generation of contamination from production machinery and personnel working in the room. If the air supply remains constant the cleanroom is dirtier if there are (a) more people in the cleanroom, (b) more activity from people, (c) cleanroom garments that are less effective in preventing dispersion of contamination, and (d) more contamination coming from production machinery and processes.

An approximation of the likely airborne cleanliness of a turbulently ventilated cleanroom can be found by use of the following equation:

$$\text{Airborne concentration (count/m}^3\text{)} = \frac{\text{Number of particles (or bacteria) generated / min}}{\text{Air volume supplied * (m}^3\text{ / min)}}$$

* including that from unidirectional flow work stations and benches

This equation cannot be used with a unidirectional flow system where the air flows in unidirectional streams, as the equation assumes that the room air is well mixed. It also assumes that the supply air is free from contamination; this is always true for the comparatively large microbe-carrying particles and true for most other particles; the exception is very small particles that can pass through the air filters.

My investigations have shown that an average person moving about with poor cleanroom garments, such as smocks or laboratory coats, can generate about 2×10^6 particles ≥ 0.5 µm/min, about 300,000 particles ≥ 5.0 µm/min, and about 160 microbe-carrying particles per minute. If people wear well-designed clothing (coverall, knee length boots, hood, etc.) made from effective fabrics the average generation of particles per minute will be about 10^6 for particles ≥ 0.5 µm, 150 000 for particles ≥ 5.0 µm and 16 for microbe-carrying particles. As discussed in Chapter 19, this will vary from person-to-person and from time-to-time. Little information is available about the generation of particles from machinery used in cleanrooms, but this can account for millions of particles ≥ 0.5 µm per minute.

By using the above equation and airborne dispersion rates, it is possible to get an estimate of the likely airborne quality of a turbulently ventilated cleanroom. Unfortunately, because of the likely lack of reliable data about the particle dispersion from the machinery and processes, it may be difficult to get an accurate result. However, as people are normally the sole source of airborne bacteria, an estimate of the airborne bacterial count will be more accurate.

5.1.2 High efficiency air filters

A cleanroom uses air filters that are much more efficient than those used in offices etc. Cleanroom filters would be normally be better than 99.97% efficient in removing particles greater than about 0.3 μm from the room's air supply. These filters are known as High Efficiency Particle Air (HEPA) filters, although Ultra Low Penetration Air (ULPA) filters, which have an even higher efficiency, are used in microelectronic fabrication and similar areas. Most cleanrooms use HEPA or ULPA filters, but in the lowest standards of cleanrooms they are not essential. In an ISO Class 8 (Class 100 000) room, bag-type filters, with an efficiency near to 90% against particles ≥ 0.5 μm, are often used.

In most cleanrooms, HEPA or ULPA filters are installed at the point where the air is discharged into the room (see Figure 5.1). In air conditioning systems in offices and the like, the filters are placed directly after the air conditioning plant and the filtered air distributed by air ducts to the air supply diffusers. However, particles may be drawn into the air supply ducts, or come off duct surfaces and hence pass into the room. The filters in cleanrooms are therefore placed in a terminal position in the air supply duct. In lower standards of cleanroom, such as ISO Class 8 (Class 100 000), the particles that could enter, or come from, the ducts will be a smaller proportion of the total count; filters are often installed in the traditional position, just after the central air conditioning plant.

5.1.3 Air movement within a turbulently ventilated cleanroom

The type, number and placement of air supply diffusers, as well as the extract grilles, is an important consideration in a turbulently ventilated cleanroom. It is possible to supply the air to a cleanroom with, or without, a diffuser. Air diffusers are used in many air conditioned rooms and situated where the supply air enters a room; they are designed to minimise the draught caused by high air velocities and ensure good air mixing. This is illustrated in Figure 5.2.

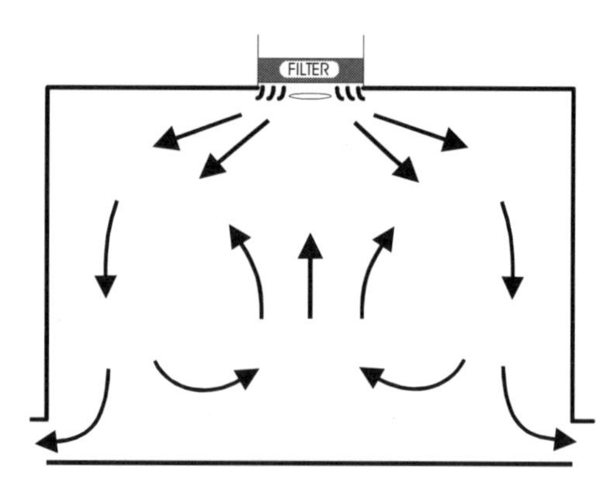

Figure 5.2 Airflow conditions produced by a ceiling diffuser

In some conventionally ventilated cleanrooms, diffusers are not used and the supply air is 'dumped' down directly from the air filter into the cleanroom. This method is chosen to obtain unidirectional flow and good contamination control conditions under the filter; it is shown diagrammatically in Figure 5.3.

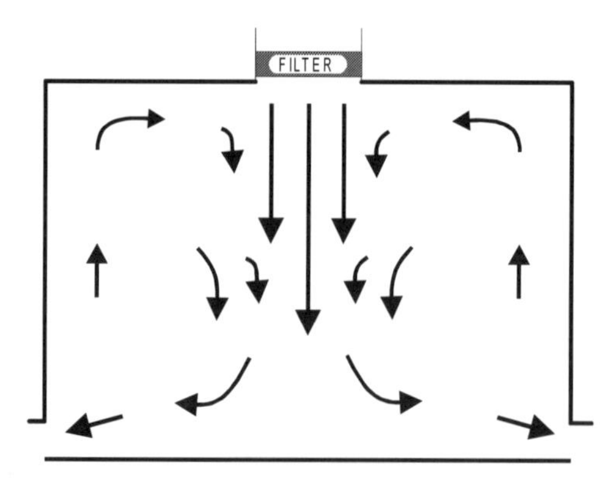

Figure 5.3 Airflow conditions produced by a 'dump' system

It is my opinion that the use of diffusers is best in conventionally ventilated cleanrooms. 'Dump' methods will give enhanced conditions below the supply area, but must therefore give poorer conditions elsewhere in the room. If enhanced conditions are required at critical areas, then it is better to ensure good air mixing in the cleanroom by means of diffusers, and use unidirectional cabinets or workstations at the critical areas. Diffusers should, however, be selected so that there are a sufficient number and size to give good mixing and draught-free conditions.

If the 'dump' method is chosen then the filters should preferably be distributed evenly about the room. There may be an advantage in grouping the filters together to protect an area that must be kept clean. However, if grouping is employed, it should be remembered that the standard of the cleanroom is determined by the dirtiest part and this may give a lower classification. Some further information on this topic is given in Section 6.1.3.

It is normal practice in cleanrooms to site the air extract grilles at a low level around the walls; it is thought that high-level extracts cause a short-circuiting of air from the air supply and hence the room is not swept by clean air. This will happen in a unidirectional flow, as the air moves in lines. However, in turbulently ventilated cleanrooms when diffusers are used, the air supply is quickly and thoroughly mixed with the rest of the room; this is the function of a diffuser. If diffusers are not used, the airflow from the filters is more unidirectional and short-circuiting to an extract is more likely to occur. Where the air extract is positioned is likely to be of little consequence if diffusers are used; in this situation any small advantage in using low level extracts is unlikely to be significant enough to require low level extracts if the design is more logical with high-level wall extracts.

5.1.4 Room pressurisation and air movement control between rooms

A cleanroom must be designed to ensure that contaminated air does not come into the room from dirtier adjacent areas. Air should therefore always move from the cleanroom to less-clean adjacent areas. In Figure 5.1 the air will move out from the central production room to both the clothing change and materials transfer areas, and onwards to the outside corridor.

To ensure that the movement is in the correct direction, airflow can be observed by smoke, water vapour or streamers; these methods are discussed in Section 11.2. However, although this method is satisfactory when setting up a cleanroom prior to hand-over, it is not a long-term monitoring possibility. To monitor a cleanroom, it is normal practice to check that the cleaner areas are more positively pressurised than less-clean adjacent areas.

If a cleanroom is at a higher pressure than an adjacent area then air will flow from the cleanroom to the adjacent area. Differential pressures of 10 Pa between two cleanrooms, and 15 Pa between a cleanroom and an unclassified area, are reasonable design pressures (12Pa = 0.05 inch water gauge). Where practical difficulties arise in achieving these pressures, e.g. where there is a supply tunnel connecting the two areas, a minimum pressure differential of 5 Pa may be acceptable.

In a cleanroom suite, the air pressures should be set up so that the air moves from clean to the less-clean areas. This means that the highest pressure should be in the production area. Figure 5.4 is a diagram of a cleanroom suite that is slightly more complicated than Figure 5.1, as it has a two rooms in the clothing change area and hence another pressure differential to be maintained. In this suite the production room would be set at a pressure of 35 Pa compared to the outside approach corridor. This is necessary to give a 10 Pa pressure difference between the production room and the clothing change room, a 10 Pa difference between the change room and locker room and 15 Pa between the locker room and the outside approach corridor; this gives a total of 35 Pa.

Because a 35 Pa pressure difference is established between the production room and the outside corridor, the same pressure is available across the material transfer room. The material transfer area can therefore be 15 Pa less than the production area and 20 Pa greater that the outside corridor; this pressure differential is greater than required but quite acceptable. However, if too large a pressure difference is used, extra energy costs will be incurred. Problems may also be experienced when trying to open and close doors, as well as 'whistling' through cracks.

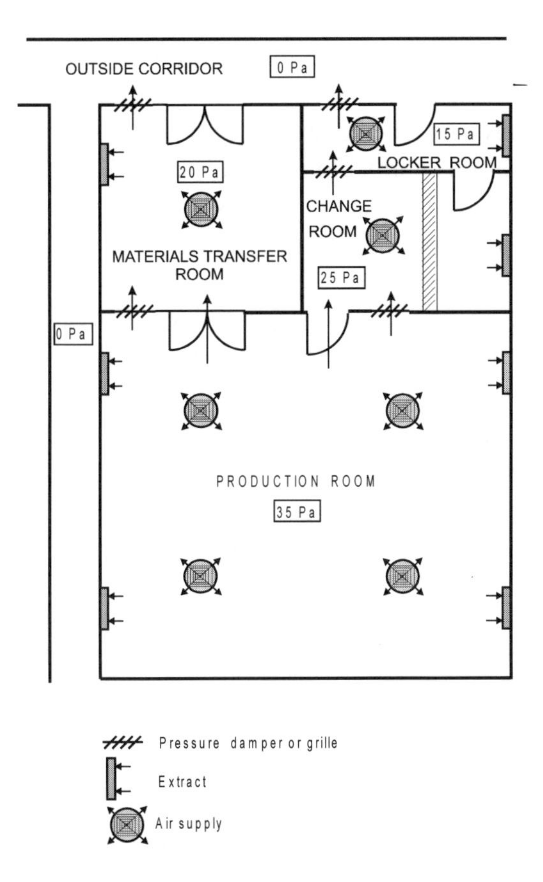

Figure 5.4 A simple cleanroom suite showing pressures and airflow between areas

It must be decided what type of air movement control scheme between rooms in the cleanroom suite should be used. Two adjacent rooms, with their door closed can be set up with just sufficient air flowing through the gaps to give the correct, differential pressure between them. This is known as the 'closed door' solution. However, the air flowing through the doorway may be quite small (especially if the door is a tight fit). The consequence of this is that when the door is opened little air is available to pass out through the doorway. There can then be an exchange of air across the open doorway caused by the air turbulence and an air temperature difference between the rooms. This may be acceptable and many cleanrooms are set up in this way. To minimise this unwanted air transfer it is normal to use an air lock, e.g. the materials transfer, or clothes changing areas. These air locks should be ventilated so that the contaminated air from the outside corridor, and any contaminants generated within the air lock can be diluted.

It may not be possible to provide an airlock between each cleanroom area, or it may be considered that the airborne contamination within an air lock is too high and should not be allowed to flow into the production area. It will then be necessary to provide an 'open door' solution, in which a system of cascading air passes through the open doorway in sufficient volume to prevent contaminated air entering.

The design used to ensure the correct airflow between rooms when the doors are open can be quite complicated. A solution to these problems is outwith the scope of this book. Readers who are interested in this topic should consult Chapter 4 of my book 'Cleanroom Design' published by John Wiley & Sons (1999).

5.1.5 Construction materials and finishes

Another indication that a room is a cleanroom is its construction method. Cleanrooms should be constructed to minimise air leakage out of the room. The internal surface finishes should also be sufficiently tough to resist chipping or powdering when impacted, or abraded. The surface finish should also be smooth, easy-to-clean and not harbour dirt in cracks. Construction materials and surface finishes are discussed further in Chapter 7 of this book.

5.2 Ancillary Cleanrooms

Adjacent to the main production cleanroom there will be other cleanrooms. The number and type of these rooms will vary according to what is being produced within the cleanroom suite and the complexity of the task. In the simple cleanroom of the type shown in Figure 5.1, it can be seen that there is a room for personnel to change their clothing, and one to bring materials in and out of the production room. In other cleanrooms there may be additional rooms to produce materials required for the production room. These may also require additional clothing change materials transfer and storage areas.

5.2.1 Clothing change area

Rooms used for changing into, and out of, cleanroom clothing vary in design. The number of rooms in the change area, and whether these rooms are divided into two or more zones by crossover benches, will vary. The design of the change areas may also be complicated if separate change rooms are provided for the two sexes. Sometimes lockers for outdoor clothing and valuables are provided outside the change area, and sometimes inside.

Figure 5.5 is a diagram showing the plan view of a one-room change area which can be either one or two zones. In this type of room, personnel come into the room, take off their excess clothing and change into cleanroom garments and exit directly into the cleanroom; all of the change procedures are carried out in the one room. A pass-over bench is often provided to divide this room into two zones. This bench provides a seat for personnel to change or cover footwear; it also divides the room into two zones of cleanliness. A single room is popular in the more economically designed cleanroom. It is also successfully used in high quality cleanrooms with high numbers of staff, and often found in the microelectronics industry. Sometimes an airlock is additionally provided to minimise the transfer of contamination from the change area into the production area.

Figure 5.6 shows three possible designs of a two-room change area; these rooms can also be further divided into zones by a pass-over bench. These rooms and zones can also be built in line. Change areas that have the greater number of rooms and zones give a more secure method of ensuring that the outside of the clothing is not contaminated, but more time has to be devoted to changing.

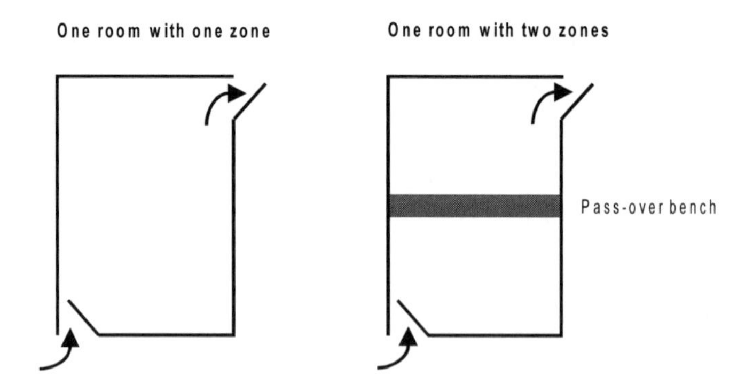

Figure 5.5 One-room change areas

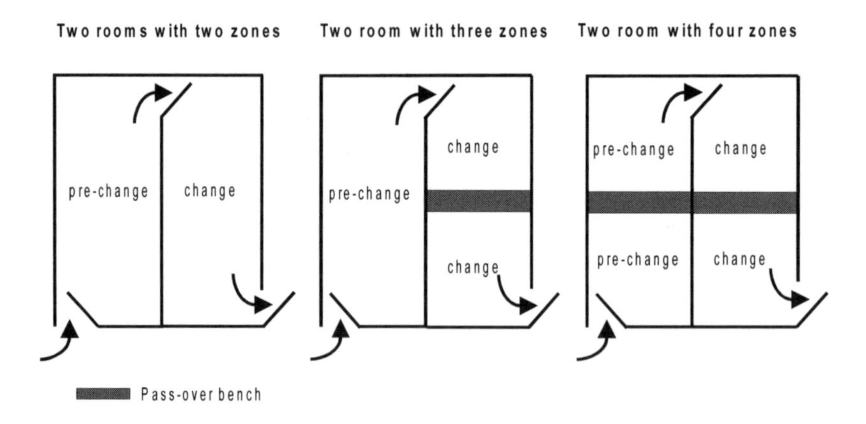

Figure 5.6 Two-room change areas with, or without, pass-over benches

Procedures used to change in and out of cleanroom clothing are discussed in detail in Chapter 19; this should be consulted for an explanation as to how these rooms are used.

Consideration should also be given to where cleanroom garments should be stored if they are used again on re-entry. They should be stored so that contamination is minimised. In higher quality cleanrooms, clothing hangers are provided in a unidirectional flow of air. An example of this method is shown in Figure 5.7.

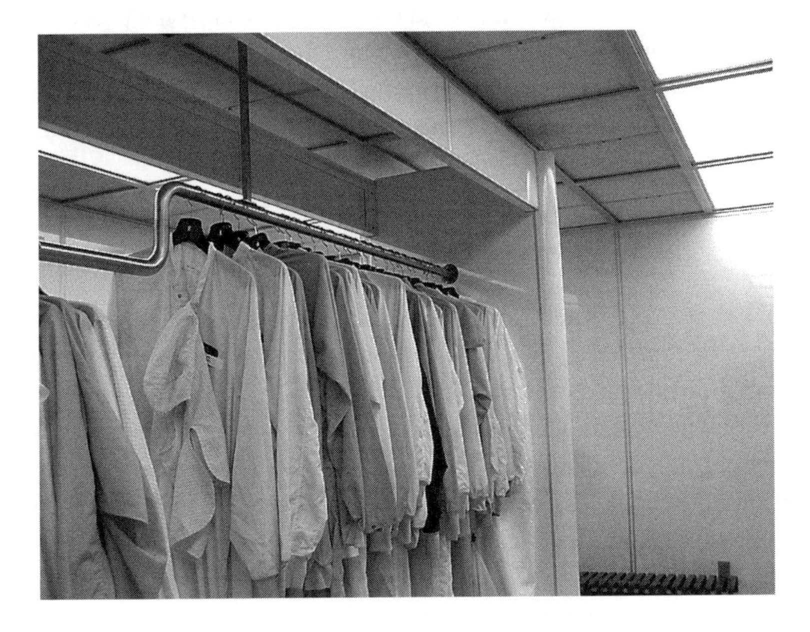

Figure 5.7 Cleanroom clothing under a vertical unidirectional airflow

Other methods require the provision of lockers, pegs for clothing bags, or pigeon holes; further information is given in Section 17.3. Some change areas, especially those where cleanroom garments are changed at every entry, have a separate area for personnel to leave the cleanroom.

Air showers are sometimes provided between the change areas and the cleanroom. Personnel enter the air shower and turn around as air jets play on their cleanroom clothing. An air shower is designed to remove particles from clothing and hence reduce dispersion in a cleanroom. However, their use is controversial. I have studied the particle dispersion from people after showering as well as the particle count in the cleanroom, and it is my opinion that air showers do little to reduce contamination in cleanrooms. However, they do have a psychological effect of reminding personnel that they are entering a special area. This benefit, however, should be balanced against the production time lost while using, or waiting to get into, the air shower.

Cleanroom flooring and mats that remove dirt from shoes should be placed on the change areas floor. Where they are placed, and the type used, varies. More information is contained in Section 17.2.1.

5.2.2 Materials transfer area

Figure 5.1 shows a typical airlock used as a materials transfer area. This allows materials to be transferred into the cleanroom with the minimum of contamination. More information as to how these are used is given in Chapter 18.

An airlock may be divided into two zones by a crossover bench. However, a bench should not be provided if it is an obstacle to large equipment that is brought into the room. The materials transfer airlock will minimise the transfer of contamination from the outside corridor to the production room, and give a clean environment suitable for unwrapping the materials transferred into the production room. It should therefore be ventilated.

Air lock doors are often interlocked to ensure that both doors cannot be opened simultaneously. This minimises the direct exchange of air from the outside corridor to the production room. Airlocks can also have indicator lights fitted outside the doors to show if anyone is in it. They ensure that when a person from the outside corridor enters the airlock, personnel from the cleanroom cannot also enter.

5.3 Containment Rooms

Cleanrooms are used to prevent the contamination of articles produced in the room. However, some manufacturing processes produce toxic chemicals or dangerous bacteria and these must be contained in a clean environment. This can occur, for example, in the pharmaceutical industry where highly active pharmaceuticals, such as hormones, must be kept clean but must not reach the operator. Other examples are found in the biotechnology industry where rooms are required to contain the genetically-engineered micro-organisms. Microbiological laboratories dealing with dangerous micro-organisms require that the personnel working in them, or the people passing near them, are not infected.

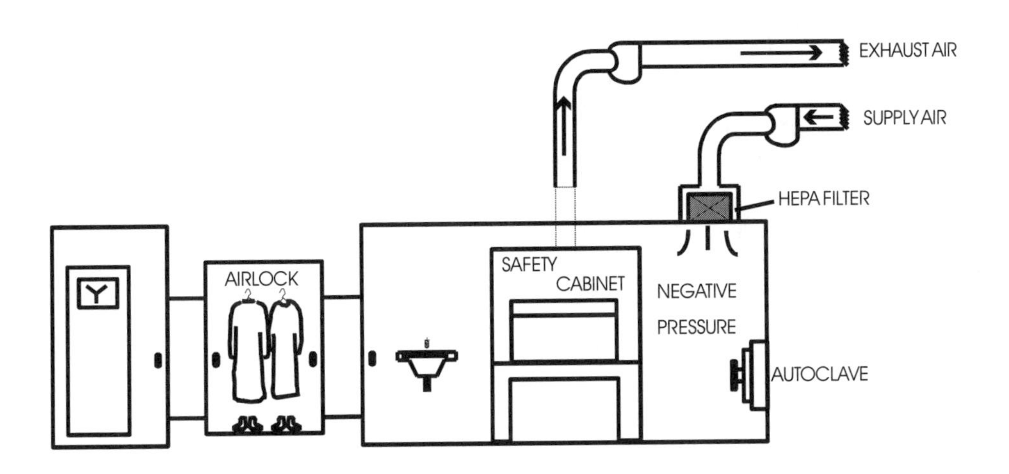

Figure 5.8 Containment room

The technology associated with the design of these containment rooms is similar to that used in cleanrooms, as containment rooms are often cleanrooms with containment facilities.

Figure 5.8 is an example of a containment room that might be used for working with micro-organisms which are dangerous to the health of the personnel working within it, or to anyone passing close to the room.

It may be seen that clean air is supplied to the room, but more air must be extracted so that the room will be under a negative pressure and air will always flow into the room. The air that is extracted must be filtered through a high efficiency filter before being discharged to the outside environment. In Figure 5.8 this is done through the safety, or containment, cabinet.

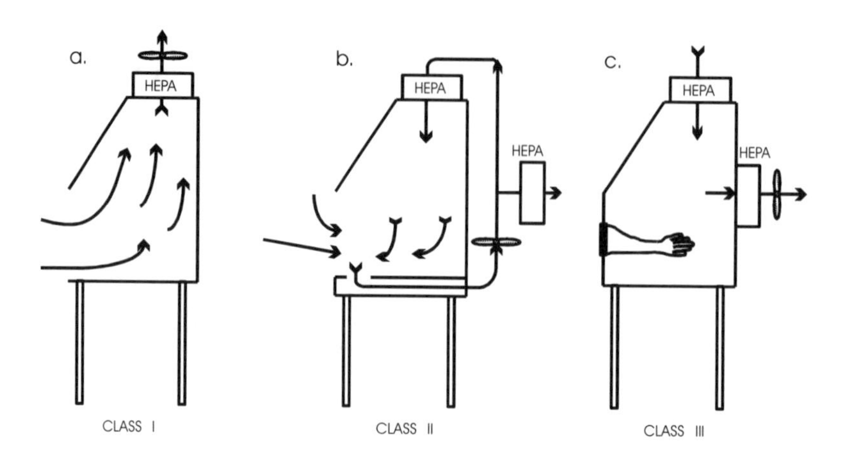

Figure 5.9 Containment cabinets

Within the containment room shown in Figure 5.8 there is likely to be a safety cabinet. Shown in Figure 5.9 is a diagrammatic representation of the three types of safety cabinets that are available, showing their airflow and isolation principles. In a room where there is not a very high safety risk, a Class I or Class II cabinet is used. If clean conditions similar to the cleanroom are acceptable, a Class I cabinet may be chosen, as this isolates contamination in it by drawing air from the room. However, if cleaner conditions than the room are required then a Class II cabinet is used; this type gives a flow of filtered air over the product, while still ensuring a flow of air into the cabinet. In a high-risk area, a Class III cabinet would be used. A Class III cabinet is very similar, if not identical, to some designs of negative-pressure isolators and an overlap in design occurs here. Negative-pressure isolators can therefore be used in such applications.

Another feature that may be found in containment rooms is an air lock to allow people to change into special clothing and to minimise airflow out of the containment room. A pass-through autoclave may be available to allow the sterilisation of contaminated material.

Other containment rooms may be of a higher or lower standard, depending on the toxic, chemical or microbiological hazard of the room. Less hazardous rooms would not use an airlock or pass-through autoclave and rely on the exhaust of a Class I cabinet to create a negative pressure in the room. Rooms in which the hazard was high would use a Class III type of cabinet or a negative pressure isolator, and may provide a shower area between the air lock and the room. In particularly hazardous situations, personnel would wear suits supplied with filtered air. Chapter 6 of my book 'Cleanroom Design' is devoted to the design of containment facilities.

Acknowledgement

Figure 5.7 is reproduced by permission of Roger Diener of Analog Devices.

6

Design of Unidirectional Cleanrooms and Clean Air Devices

Cleanrooms that are ventilated in the turbulent manner described in the previous chapter may achieve conditions as low as ISO Class 6 (Class 1000) during manufacturing, but this is more likely to be ISO Class 7 (Class 10 000). To obtain rooms better than ISO Class 6 (Class 1000) during operation, greater dilution of the generated particles is required. This can be achieved by a unidirectional flow of air.

6.1 Unidirectional Cleanrooms

Unidirectional airflow is used in cleanrooms when low airborne concentrations of particles or micro-organisms is required. This type of cleanroom was previously known as 'laminar flow', both names describing the flow of air. The airflow is in one direction, either horizontal or vertical, at a uniform speed that is normally between 0.3 and 0.5 m/s (60 ft/min to 100 ft/min) and throughout the entire air space. Figure 6.1 is a cross-section through a typical vertical flow type of cleanroom. It may be seen that air is supplied from a complete bank of high efficiency filters in the roof of the cleanroom. The air then flows down through the room like an air piston, thus removing the contamination. It then exits through the floor, mixes with some fresh air brought in from outside, and recirculates back to the high efficiency air filters.

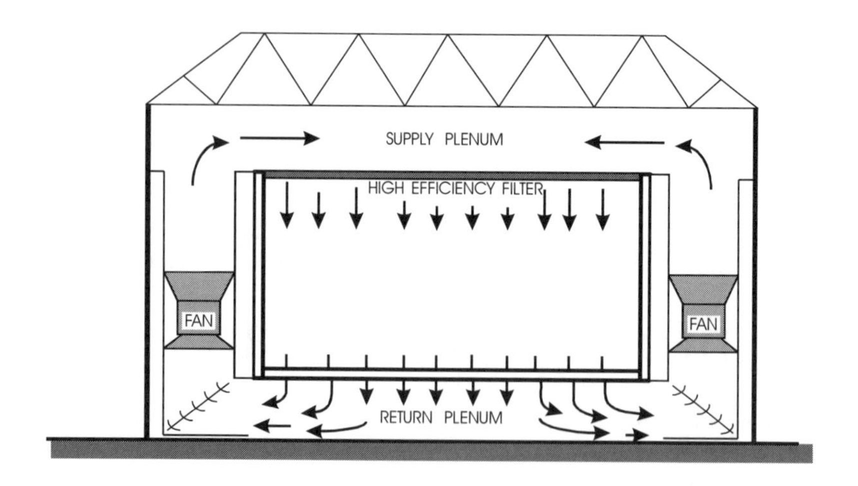

Figure 6.1 Vertical unidirectional flow cleanroom

Airborne contamination from people and processes can be immediately removed by this flow of air, whereas the turbulently ventilated system relies on mixing and dilution. In an empty room with no obstructions to the unidirectional airflow, contamination can be quickly removed by air velocities much lower than those mentioned above. However, in an operating room there are machines causing obstructions to the airflow, and people moving about it. Obstructions may cause the unidirectional flow to be turned into turbulent flow and local air recirculation to be established round the obstructions. Movement of people will also turn the unidirectional flow into turbulent flow. With lower air velocities and air dilution, higher concentration of contamination can be established in these turbulent areas. A velocity in the region of 0.3 m/s to 0.5 m/s (60 ft/min to 100 ft/min) is necessary so that disrupted unidirectional flow can be quickly reinstated and the contamination in turbulent areas round obstructions adequately diluted.

I have studied the effect of velocity in a variable-velocity unidirectional flow room that was operational. The velocity could be varied from 0.1 m/s to 0.6 m/s (20 ft/min to 120 ft/min). The results showed that a velocity of 0.3 m/s (60 ft/min) was required to give stable unidirectional flow and low particle and bacterial concentrations. Increasing the air velocity, in stages up to 0.6 m/s (120 ft/min) gave lower airborne counts, but this worked on the 'law of diminished returns'. The information obtained can be interpreted as suggesting that a velocity of 0.3 m/s (60 ft/min) gives the best returns for effort, but if a cleanroom has a high density of machinery, or personnel, a higher velocity would give lower airborne contamination.

Unidirectional airflow is correctly defined in terms of air velocity as the higher the velocity the cleaner the room. Air changes per hour are related to the volume of the room, e.g. ceiling height and are therefore incorrect units of measurement.

The air supplied to unidirectional flow rooms is many times greater (10s or 100s of times) than that supplied to a turbulently ventilated room. These cleanrooms are therefore very much more expensive to build and run.

Unidirectional flow rooms are of two general types, namely horizontal or vertical flow. In the horizontal system, the airflow is from wall to wall and in the vertical system it is from ceiling to floor.

6.1.1 Vertical flow unidirectional cleanrooms

A vertical flow unidirectional cleanroom is shown in Figure 6.1. This shows the air flowing through the complete area of a floor. However, unidirectional flow rooms are also designed so that air is returned through extract grilles distributed around the wall at floor level. This type is illustrated in Figure 6.2. This design can only be used in rooms that are not too wide, and 6 metres (20 ft) has been suggested as a maximum width.

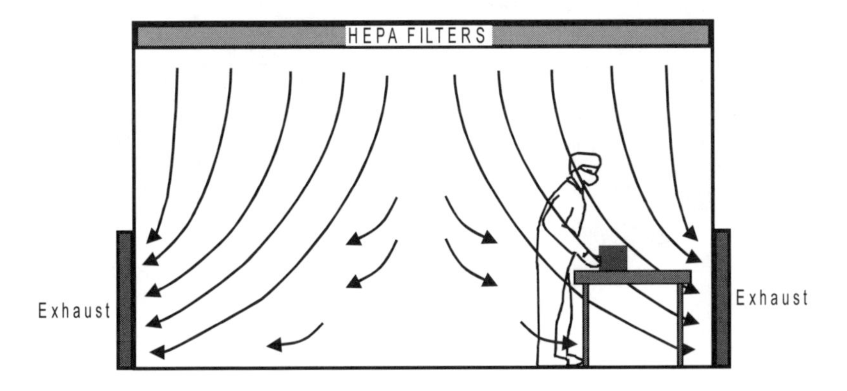

Figure 6.2 Vertical unidirectional cleanroom with exhausts in the wall

Care must be taken with this design. The route that the supply air takes to get to the air exhausts is the reason for the problem. Airflow of the type shown in Figure 6.2 gives poor unidirectional flow in the centre of the room and a flow of air that is not vertical in the rest. Personnel may therefore contaminate the product if they are positioned between the air supply and the product.

6.1.2 *Horizontal flow unidirectional flow rooms*

Figure 6.3 shows a typical design of a horizontal flow cleanroom. In this design, the air is supplied through a wall of high efficiency filters and flows across the room and exits on the other side. The air is then returned to a ventilation plant and back through the air filters. The area of a wall in most rooms is usually much smaller than the ceiling, and hence a crossflow room will cost less in capital and running costs than a downflow one. The horizontal flow type of cleanroom is not as popular as the vertical type. The reason for this is illustrated in Figure 6.4, which shows the problem that can occur with a contamination source.

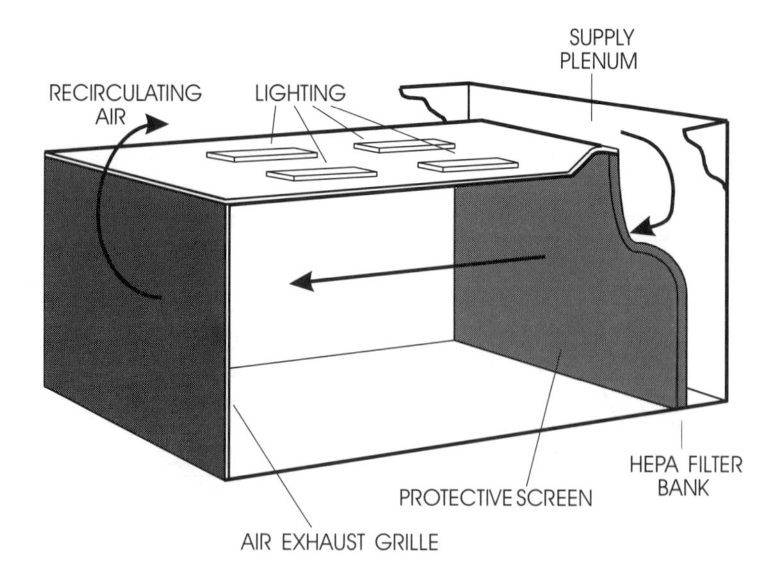

Figure 6.3 Horizontal unidirectional flow cleanrooms

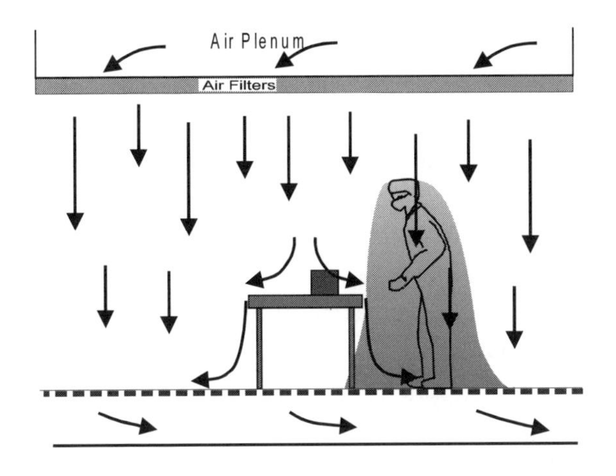

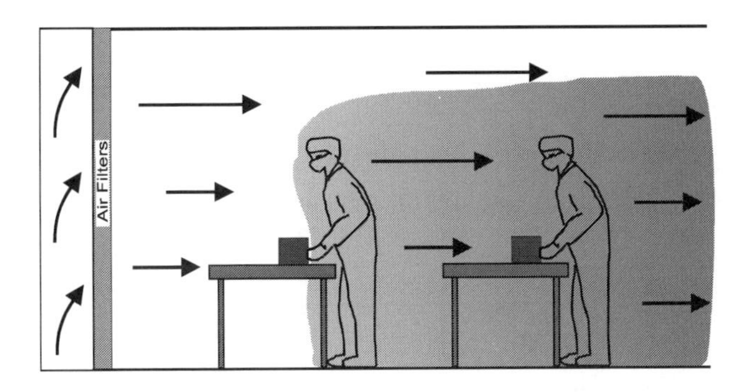

Figure 6.4 Dispersion in both a downflow and crossflow cleanroom

Any contamination generated close to the filters in a vertical flow will be swept across the room and could contaminate work that is progressing downwind. Generally speaking, a vertical flow of air gives better contamination control (as shown in Figure 6.4) because the dispersed contamination is less likely to reach the product.

If the crossflow cleanroom can be arranged so that the most critical operations are close to the supply filters and the dirtier ones at the exhaust end, then this type of room can be successful. The following works well:

1. A faulty component, requiring repair, enters the end of the room away from the filters.
2. The component is dismantled in stages as work progresses towards the filters.
3. The most susceptible-to-contamination repair is carried out next to the supply filters.
4. The component is reassembled and then packaged on its way back up the other side of the cleanroom.
5. The repaired component exits out of the room, on the opposite side from the entering components.

A crossflow type of cleanroom can also be successful if the machine or process is placed close to the filter bank and no-one passes between the filter bank and machine when production is going on.

6.1.3 Unidirectional flow rooms used in semiconductor manufacturing

Unidirectional flow cleanrooms are much used in semiconductor fabrication where the very best cleanroom conditions are required.

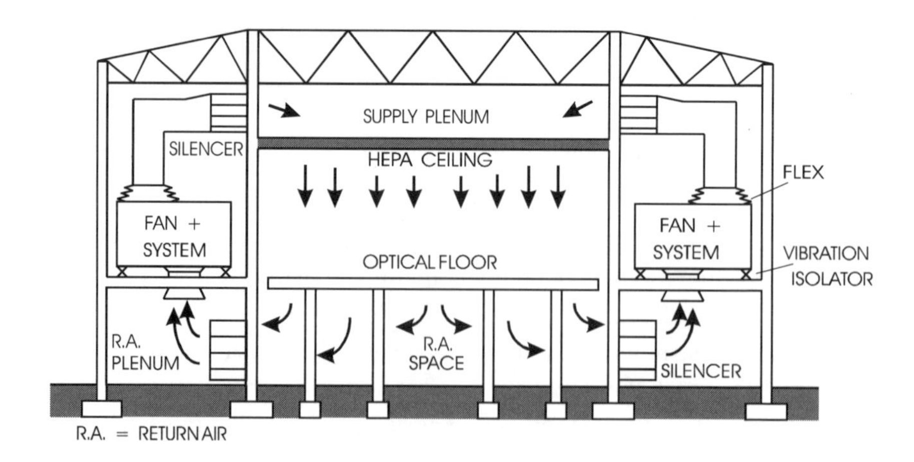

Figure 6.5 Vertical flow cleanroom often used in semiconductor manufacturing

The design of semiconductor cleanrooms has evolved over several years, but a design that has been popular for a number of years is shown in Figure 6.5. The air in Figure 6.5 flows in a unidirectional way from a ceiling of high efficiency filters and down through the floor of the cleanroom. As the manufacturing of semiconductors is sensitive to vibration, and anti-vibration measures are incorporated. Some designs return the air from just below the floor, while other designs (similar to the type shown in Figure 6.5) use a large basement, that basement being used for services. Other designs have both the sub floor and a basement below. The design shown in Figure 6.5 is often called a 'ballroom' type because there is one large cleanroom. Typically, it is over 1000 m^2 in floor area and some rooms are large enough to hold two football fields. It is expensive to run but adaptable. Figure 6.6 shows a photograph of a typical 'ballroom' cleanroom before production equipment was installed.

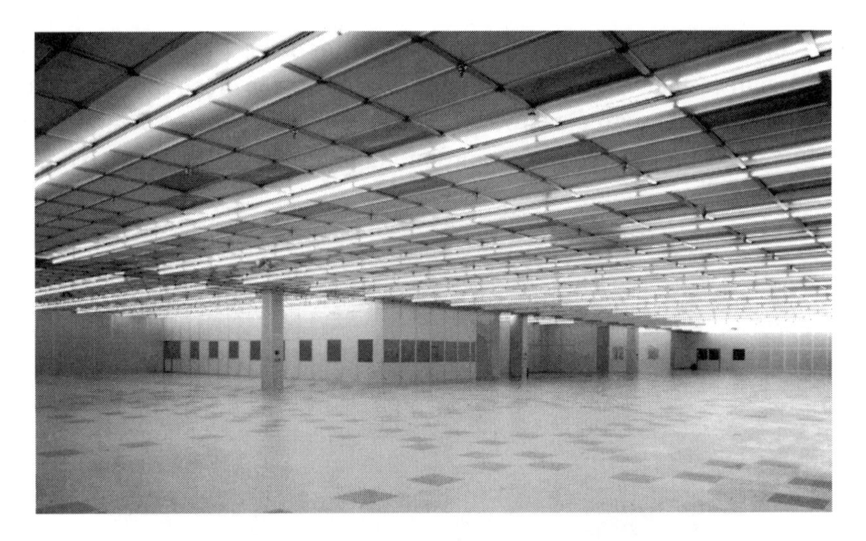

Figure 6.6 Ballroom type of cleanroom

In the 'ballroom' type of cleanroom, a complete ceiling of high efficiency filters provide clean air throughout the whole room, irrespective of need, and the machinery stands throughout the room. However, the best quality air is only really necessary where the product is exposed to airborne contamination, and lesser quality should be acceptable in other areas.

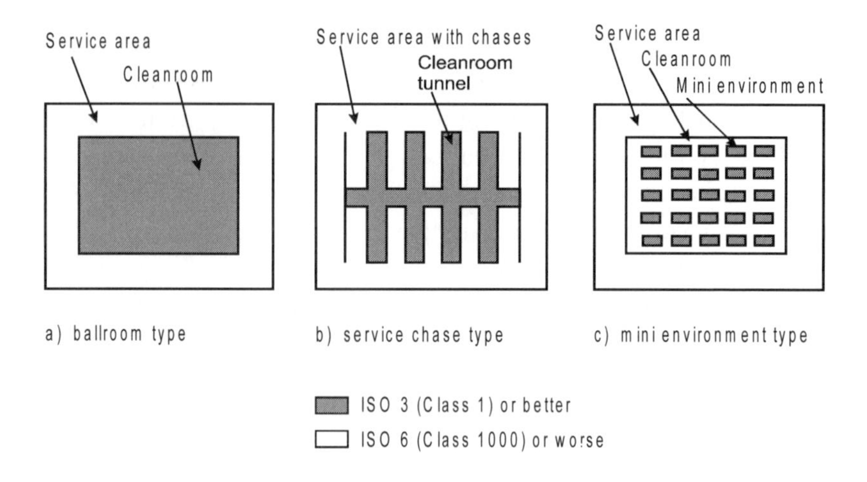

Figure 6.7 Plan views of three types of cleanrooms

Using this concept, less expensive cleanrooms have been designed. One such design is that where service chases with lower cleanliness standards are inter-dispersed with cleanroom tunnels. This concept is shown in Figure 6.7 (b), and a photograph of a cleanroom tunnel is shown in Figure 6.8.

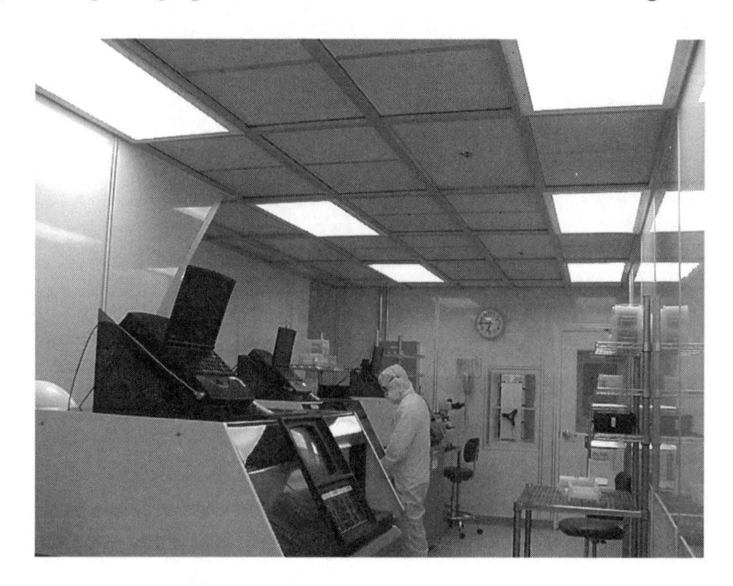

Figure 6.8 Cleanroom tunnel design

Service technicians can gain access to bulkhead-fitted machinery through the service chases without entering the clean space where the semiconductor wafers are exposed. Less expensive air conditions are provided in these service chases.

It is also possible in the ballroom type of design to divide up the 'ballroom' with prefabricated walls and provide clean tunnel and service chases; these walls can be dismantled and reassembled in a different configuration should the need arise.

Service chases and other less critical areas of the cleanroom are normally supplied with lesser quantities of air and have a lower standard of air cleanliness. This can be achieved by reducing the ceiling filter coverage by means of ceiling blanks; this method is shown diagrammatically in Figure 6.9. If this method is used, it is best to distribute the filters evenly around the ceiling. If the filters are grouped together in lines or rectangles the area under the filters will be better, but away from them will be poorer. As the cleanroom classification is determined by the poorest particle count this design may result in a poorer classification. Another alternative is to use 100% filter coverage and reduce the overall air velocity. This design is likely to give better air movement that a filter ceiling with less than 100% coverage and hence will give lower particle counts. However, it will be more expensive to build.

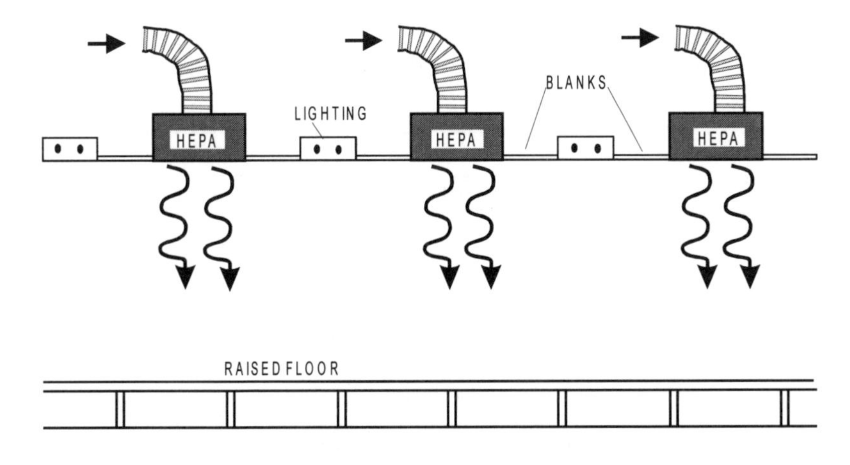

Figure 6.9 Reduced ceiling filter coverage to give non-unidirectional conditions

If either of these two methods is employed, use may be made of Table 6.1 to calculate the percentage of filter coverage. Table 6.1 is published in the Recommended Practice RP CC012 of the IEST, although the nomenclature of the room classification has been changed to that used in this book. It should be noted that 100 ft/min = 0.5 m/s, approximately.

Table 6.1 Air velocities in cleanrooms

Class of cleanroom	Airflow type	Average velocity (ft/min)	Air changes/hr
ISO 8 (100,000)	N/M	1-8	5-48
ISO 7 (10,000)	N/M	10-15	60-90
ISO 6 (1,000)	N/M	25-40	150-240
ISO 5 (100)	U/N/M	40-80	240-480
ISO 4 (10)	U	50-90	300-540
ISO 3 (1)	U	60-90	360-540
better than ISO 3	U	60-100	360-600

$$\text{Air changes per hour} = \frac{\text{Average airflow velocity}^{*} \times \text{room area} \times 60\ \text{min / hr}}{\text{Room Volume}}$$

* taken over the whole supply ceiling
N = nonunidirectional; M = mixed flow room ; U = unidirectional flow.

The values used in Table 6.1 should only be used as a guide and I consider that too much air is required to achieve the cleanroom classifications in non-unidirectional room conditions.

If the cleanroom design uses an air supply plenum then the unfiltered air in the plenum above the filters will be at a higher pressure than the air in the cleanroom. Unfiltered air can therefore leak from the supply plenum into the cleanroom through badly sealed, or unsealed, joints in the structure. This problem is discussed in Chapter 11 and shown in Figure 11.1. Such problems can be overcome if the area above the ceiling is below the pressure of the cleanroom. This can be achieved by individually supplying the filter housings with ducted air, or by using individual fan-filter modules. These methods are often used when the filter coverage is less than 100%.

6.2 Clean Air Devices

Clean air devices are used in cleanrooms to provide a higher quality of air to critical areas where products or processes are open to contamination. Types of enhanced clean air devices that are available are: unidirectional flow benches, unidirectional flow work stations, isolators and minienvironments. The use of clean air devices in a turbulently ventilated room is popular, and is the most common configuration of cleanroom. By this method, the best air conditions are provided only where they are needed and considerable cost savings are made compared to providing a full unidirectional cleanroom.

6.2.1 Unidirectional air devices

Figure 6.10 is a drawing of a horizontal flow cabinet; this is one of the simplest and most effective methods of controlling contamination.

The operator sits at the bench and works on materials, or at a process, placed on the bench top. The operator's contamination is thus kept downwind of the critical process.

Also available are a variety of styles of unidirectional flow systems that may vary in size to encompass any size of production machinery. Figure 6.11 shows a vertical flow unidirectional work station placed over a filling machine. The airflow in the cleanroom is turbulent but the product is protected from contamination by being filled in a unidirectional flow of air.

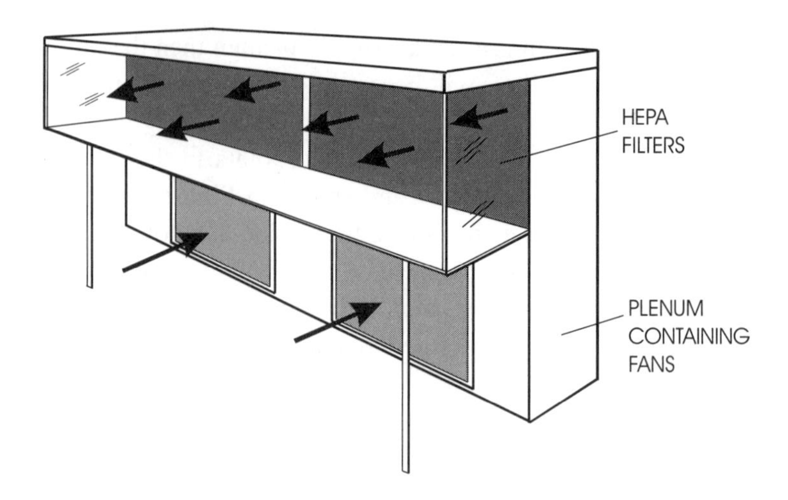

Figure 6.10 Horizontal flow cabinet

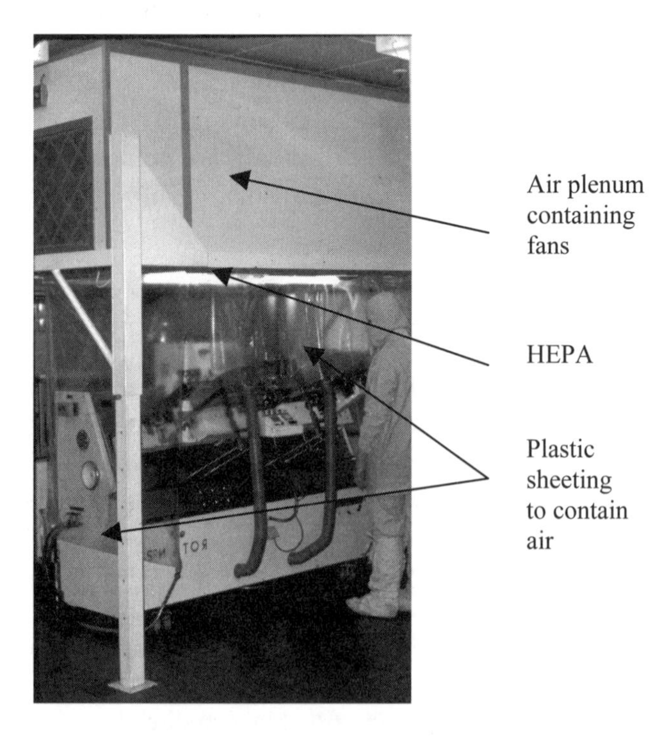

Figure 6.11 Vertical flow work station over production machinery

6.2.2 Isolators and minienvironments

A reduction in capital and running costs of a cleanroom is always sought, especially if this can be accompanied by an increase in product yield brought about by enhanced contamination control. There has therefore been much use of what have been variously called 'isolators', 'barrier technology' and 'minienvironments'. Minienvironments is the term commonly used in the semiconductor industry, the other two words are used mainly in the pharmaceutical industry.

6.2.2.1 Semiconductor applications

A minienvironment uses a physical barrier (usually plastic sheet or glass) to isolate the critical manufacturing area and provide it with the very best quality of air. The rest of the room can then be provided with lower quantities of air.

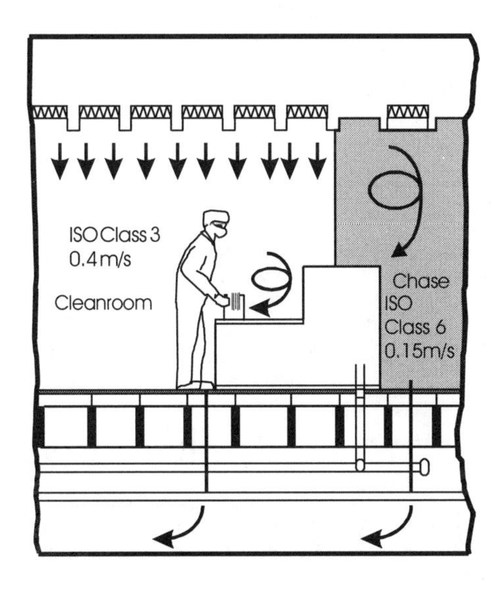

Figure 6.12 Design of unidirectional system with service chase

Figure 6.12 is a diagram of the air supply design *without* a minienvironment. In this design, large quantities of a unidirectional flow of air are provided to give the best conditions (shown as white in Figure 6.12 and designated ISO Class 3) in those parts of the room where the operators move silicon wafers from machine to machine. Lesser quantities of air are provided for the service chases where the bulkhead-fitted machines are serviced (shaded area and designated ISO Class 6).

Figure 6.13 is a diagram of an air supply design that uses minienvironments. The minienvironment (shown as white and designated as ISO Class 3) then provides the highest quality of environment. A lesser quality of environment (ISO Class 6, or poorer) is provided in both the production areas and the service chase. The total air supply volume is much less with this minienvironment design (see also Figure 6.6).

It is seen in Figure 6.13 that the air velocity in the minienvironment is shown as 0.4 m/s (80 ft/min). This is the speed associated with low particle counts in occupied cleanrooms. However, there are no personnel within the minienvironment causing turbulence and if the machinery is not giving off disruptive thermal up-currents then a lower air velocity may suffice. The minimum velocity that is suitable will have to be determined by use of air visualisation techniques described in Section 11.2.

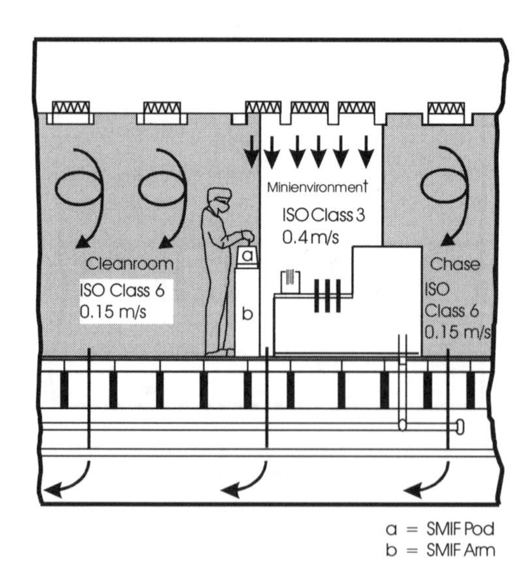

Figure 6.13 Semiconductor fabrication room with a SMIF isolation system

As well as using a minienvironment to isolate the area where the silicon wafers are exposed, the wafers can also be transported between processing machines in specially designed carriers (SMIF Pods), which prevent the wafers being contaminated by the air outside. These pods are slotted into the machine through a Standard Mechanical Interface Format (SMIF). The wafers are processed and then loaded back into a carrier; it is detached and taken to another machine and loaded into its interface. The transfer of the carrier is usually done by a person but automatic handling systems are also used.

Various types of minienvironments, with different methods of accessing the wafers into the production machines, have been developed. As long as these are well designed, particularly with respect to the container for the wafer cassettes and the transfer port, they will work well.

6.2.2.2 Other cleanroom applications

Isolator and barrier technology has been applied successfully to pharmaceutical and other types of manufacturing. They can be used to either protect the product from contamination, personnel from toxic compounds, or in some cases, both. Isolators can be purchased with various design attributes. Some of these design attributes are shown in Figure 6.14.

Design attributes of an isolator that should be considered are as follows:

- whether they are positively or negatively pressurised with respect to the room they are situated;
- the type of transfer systems for the entry and exit of materials;
- methods to be used for manipulating inside the isolator.

The cleanliness of the product, or process, inside an isolator will be maintained by using a positively pressurised isolator. Internal pressures in the order of 20 to 70 Pa, compared to the surroundings, are typical. Where hazard containment is required, a negative pressure system is used.

The type of transfer device selected for transferring items in and out of an isolator will greatly influence its efficiency. Figure 6.14 shows both a pass-through sterilising tunnel and a transfer-docking device.

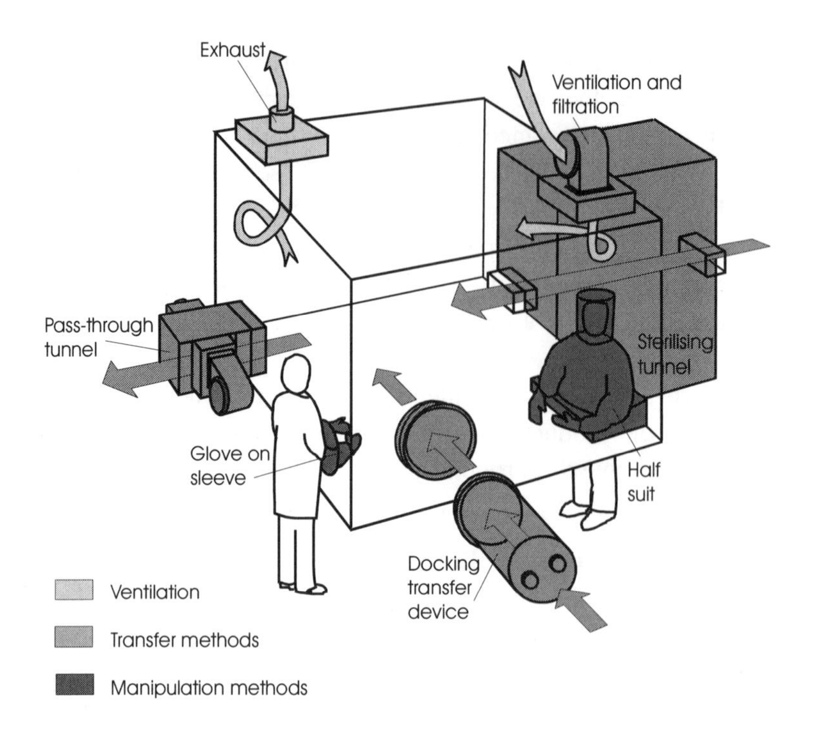

Figure 6.14 An isolator with its various components

Docking devices are the most efficient method of ensuring that the materials pass into an isolator without being contaminated. They may also be used to connect or separate individual isolators. The sequence shown in figure 6.15 illustrates the operating principles of a typical transfer device. This docking port method is the most secure, but it is not the easiest method of manipulating materials in and out of an isolator. Other simpler methods are available.

A transfer hatch, or pass box, can be used where the manufacturing or testing, is being carried out in batches. Figure 6.16 illustrates an isolator with transfer hatch, or pass box, on each side. These can be provided with an appropriate combination of interlocked doors and ventilation.

When the manufacturing process is continuous, as with large scale manufacturing, then it is more convenient if the product can be continually transferred out of the isolator. This can be by either using a final holding isolator and one of the methods described above. A aerodynamically designed 'mouse hole' or transfer tunnel, can be used together with an outward flow of air (see Figure 6.14).

Most isolators require people to manipulate products within the isolators. This is achieved by the use of glove ports or half suits. These two methods are illustrated in Figure 6.14. Figure 6.17 also shows the inside of an isolator and two operators working with half suits.

Step 1
Container (or transport isolator) approaches closed isolator port.

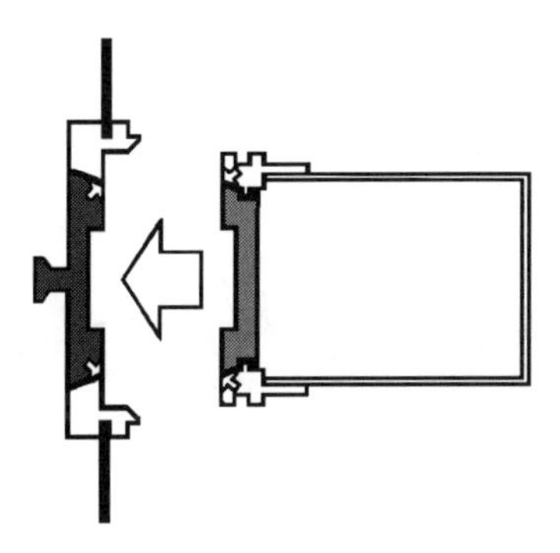

Step 2
Container docks with port and rotates to lock and enclose exposed faces. At the same time the interlock is released on the isolator door.

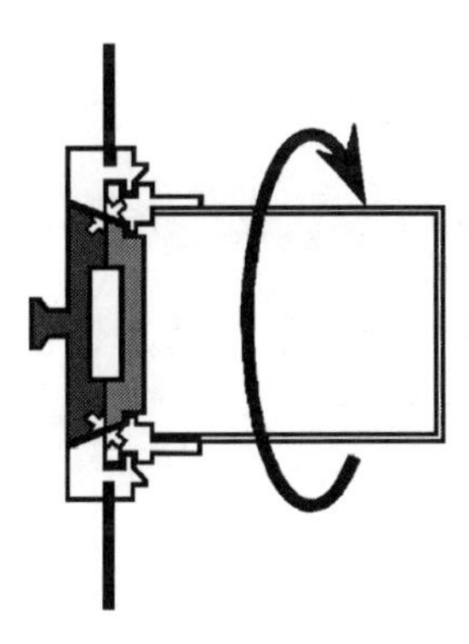

Step 3
Door into isolator is opened to allow free communication between the two enclosed volumes.

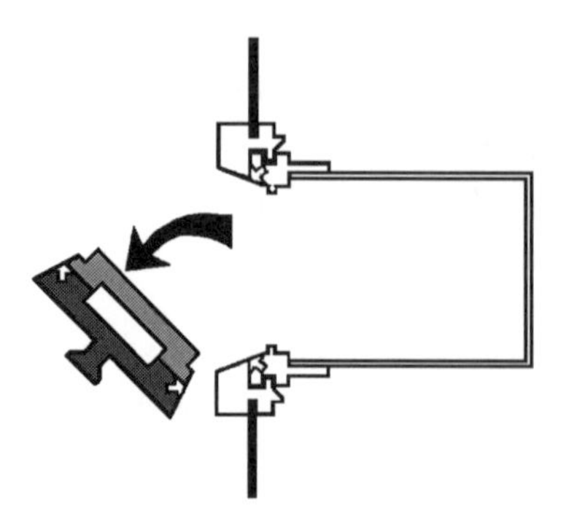

Figure 6.15 Operation of a transfer port

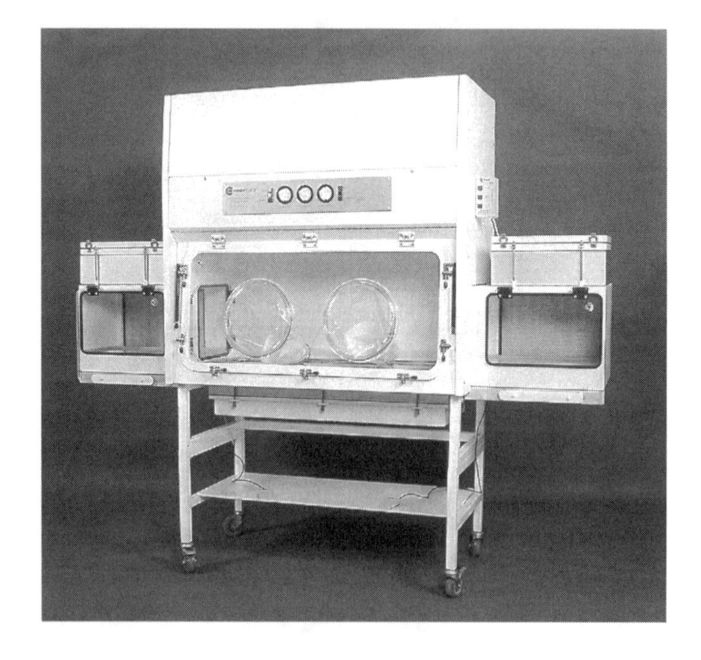

Figure 6.16 Photograph of an isolator with transfer chambers

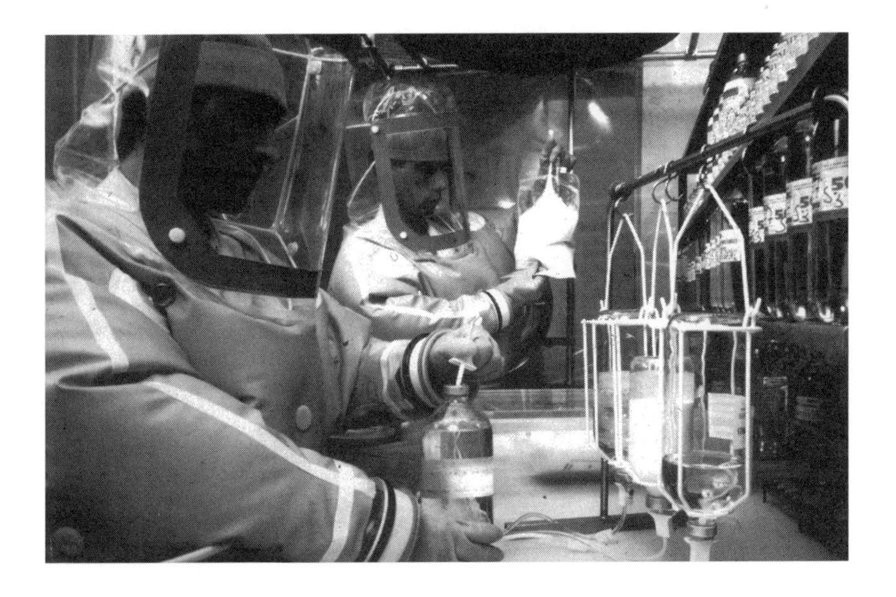

Figure 6.17 View of half suits and inside of isolator

Acknowledgements

Figures 6.5 and 6.9 are reproduced by permission of Gordon King. Figure 6.6 is reproduced by permission of M+W Pearce. Figure 6.8 is reproduced by permission of Roger Diener of Analog Devices. Figures 6.12 and 6.13 are reproduced by permission of Asyst Technologies. Figures 6.14, 6.15 and 6.17 are reproduced by permission of La Calhene. Figure 6.16 is reproduced by permission of Envair. Table 6.1 is reproduced by permission of the Institute of Environmental Sciences and Technology.

7

Construction Materials and Surface Finishes

7.1 General Requirements

A cleanroom requires a higher standard of construction than many other buildings. Construction materials used to build cleanrooms differ from those used in non-cleanroom construction for the following reasons:

- A cleanroom should be built with an airtight structure.
- The internal surface finish should be smooth and suitable for cleaning.
- The internal surface finish should be sufficiently tough to resist chipping or powdering when impacted or abraded.
- Some process chemicals, cleaning agents, disinfectants and water may attack or penetrate conventional finishes.
- In some cleanrooms, electro-dissipative construction materials will be required.
- In some cleanrooms, construction materials that give a minimum of 'outgassing' will be required.

Cleanrooms are maintained at a positive pressure with respect to adjacent areas. If the construction is poor and the joints not well sealed, then the structure may leak too much. It may then be necessary to pressurise the room by excessive amounts of 'make up' outside air. It is not good economic sense to waste air that has to be expensively filtered and air-conditioned. Attempting to seal up the structure during the 'snagging' part of the construction will not be as successful as making it airtight during construction. Containment rooms that are maintained at a negative pressure must be airtight, as dirty unfiltered air will be drawn into the room through cracks, joints and at service penetration points in the fabric.

The materials that are used for the construction of a cleanroom should be smooth on the surface facing the inside of the cleanroom. There should be no pores or roughness that will retain contamination. The surface should be free of ledges and easily wiped free of any contamination that is deposited. The butts and joints, as seen from the inside of the cleanroom, should not show openings that may harbour, and then disperse, dirt.

The surface finish in a cleanroom must not break up easily and disperse chips or particles of material. A conventional material that is often used in houses and offices is plasterboard that is nailed to stud partitions and then painted. If this material is struck heavily the plaster powder will be released. This is unacceptable in a cleanroom and surface finishes must be suitably resistant to impact.

Cleanroom surfaces, especially floors, should be able to withstand liquids used in cleanrooms. Some processes use strong acids or solvents that will attack surfaces. Cleanrooms, where micro-organisms cause contamination, will require disinfection. Disinfectants are in an aqueous solution and to correctly disinfect the surface the contact time should be several minutes; water penetration can occur if construction materials are not suitable. Similar problems can occur when cleaning the cleanroom with surfactant solutions. It is therefore necessary to ensure that penetration of water does not occur, as this can produce conditions that are suitable for microbial growth. It should, however, be noted that it is incorrect to suggest that micro-organisms sitting in dry conditions in cracks and pores will multiply. Micro-organisms are aquatic in nature, and unless free water is available, or the relative humidity is very much higher than found in a cleanroom, growth will not occur.

An electrostatic charge can be generated by rubbing two dissimilar surfaces together and can give two problems. Firstly, the charge will attract particles from the air and those deposited particles may give a contamination problem. Secondly, electrostatic discharge can cause some components to fail. Construction materials that minimise this problem may be necessary in some cleanrooms.

Some chemicals can 'outgas' from the materials used in construction of cleanrooms. These outgassed chemicals are often called 'molecular contamination'. In some cleanrooms, such as those required for manufacturing optical surfaces or semiconductors, the deposition of these materials onto the product may be unacceptable. Where this is a problem, construction materials that do not outgas will be required.

Cleanrooms can be constructed in various ways. However, despite the fact that some construction methods will not fit easily into either group, the building techniques can be discussed under two headings: conventional and modular. These are discussed below.

7.2 Conventional Building Techniques

Conventional building techniques, suitably modified, can be used in cleanroom construction. The building used to house the cleanroom suite will be conventionally constructed with floor, ceiling and external walls. Inside that structure, internal walls will become the various rooms of the cleanroom suite. These are constructed using conventional techniques employing bricks or blocks and finished using wet plastering or dry lining methods.

The dry finishing method is the most popular method as this employs less site time, is more easily repaired and allows the electricity, and other services such as air ducts to be run behind. At its simplest, wall studs are used and these are lined with plasterboard. The boards are taped, primed and painted. The paint is sprayed on and will be chosen to give good impact resistance, e.g. epoxy-based types. To assist cleaning, wall-to-wall corners are best constructed with 25 mm (1 inch) to 50 mm (2 inch) diameter curves. The corner where the wall meets the floor would normally be finished with a 100 mm (4 inch) quarter-round coving. If this method is used, it would only be suitable for lightly-used cleanrooms of about ISO Class 8 (Class 100 000), or for approach corridors or controlled areas outside the cleanroom.

A considerable improvement in the quality of the cleanroom can be achieved by lining the frames with various sheets of cleanroom-compatible material; this will also enhance the look of the cleanroom.

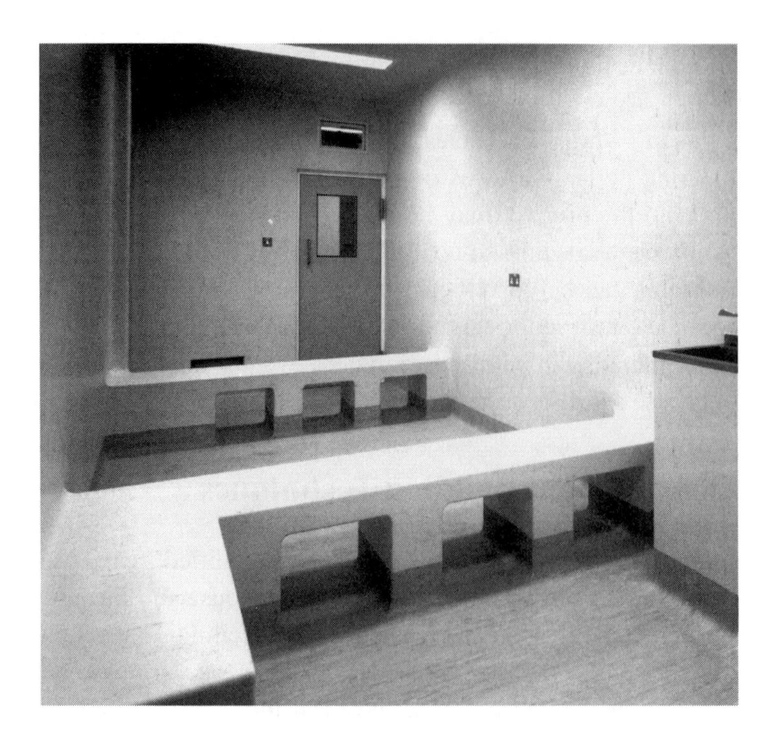

Figure 7.1 Cleanroom change area showing good use of curves

The panels will be thinner – from about 3mm to 12 mm (1/8 inch to ½ inch) depending on their strength and rigidity – than the studless system used in modular construction because the frames will give additional rigidity.
The following wall panels can be used:

- Panels laminated with an outer cleanroom-compatible surface and an inner-strengthening core. Outer surfaces can be (a) mild steel that is galvanised and either powder coated or enamelled, (b) plastic sheets or (c) aluminium that is either anodised, powder coated or enamelled. Inner core materials can be plaster, composite board, plywood, honeycombing, etc.;
- Glass-reinforced epoxy sheets;
- Mild steel sheets that are galvanised and either powder coated or enamelled;

- Aluminium sheets that are anodised, powder coated or enamelled;
- Stainless steel sheets, with or without a suitable paint finish.

Many other combinations and materials can be used, as long as they fulfil the criteria defined in the first section of this chapter.

7.3 Modular Construction

Modular construction is the type of construction where components are delivered ready-made and assembled on site. A large variety of modular components are available from firms who specialise in manufacturing such systems. Inevitably, the most easily assembled, best looking and most robust system, with the least likelihood of contamination problems, will be the most expensive. It is therefore necessary to choose wisely, balancing the quality and cost of the products with the advantages they bring. The two principal ways a modular system are assembled are:

- Studless wall systems
- Framed wall constructions.

7.3.1 Studless wall systems

These are normally assembled from wall panels that are about 50 mm (2 inch) thick for rigidity; these are slotted into ceiling and floor mounted tracks. These tracks are usually anodised aluminium extrusions and the wall panels are butted together. Figure 7.2 shows a drawing of the ceiling and floor details of a high quality system of this type. Figure 7.3 shows ceiling and floor details of a less expensive system of this type.

The wall panels are laminated from an outer cleanroom compatible surface and inner-strengthening core. Outer surfaces can be plastic sheets, aluminium that is either anodised, powder coated or enamelled, and suitably treated mild steel. Inner core materials can be plaster, composite board, plywood, honeycombing, etc.

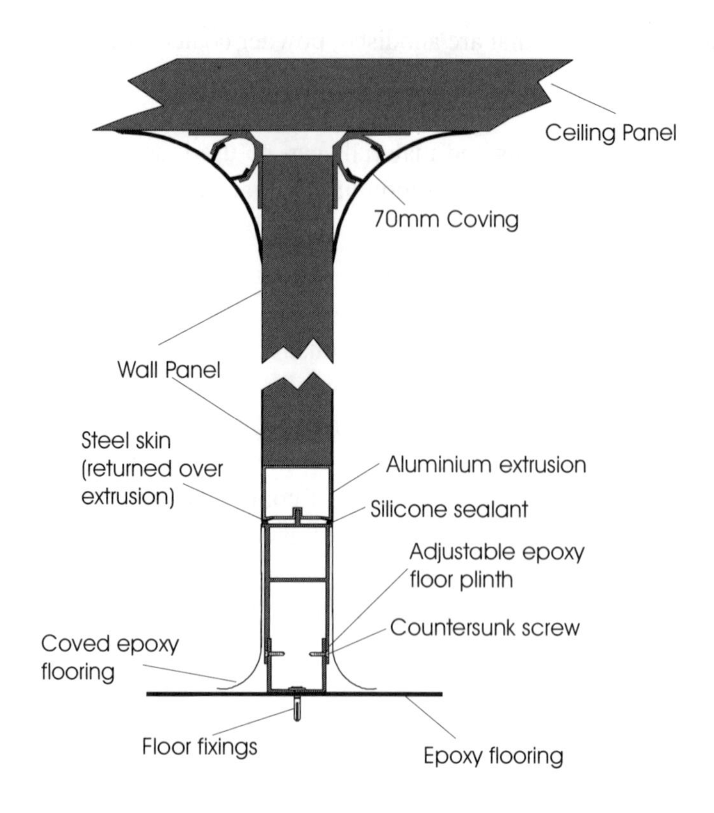

Figure 7.2 Cross-section of ceiling and floor details of high quality modular system

7.3.2 Framed wall systems

These systems are built from joined aluminium extrusions. If this method is used for a room, the studs and cross members are clad with wall panels either on one side (single shell) or on both (double shells). Wall panels used in this type of construction will be made of the same types of materials as discussed above, although they will be thinner.

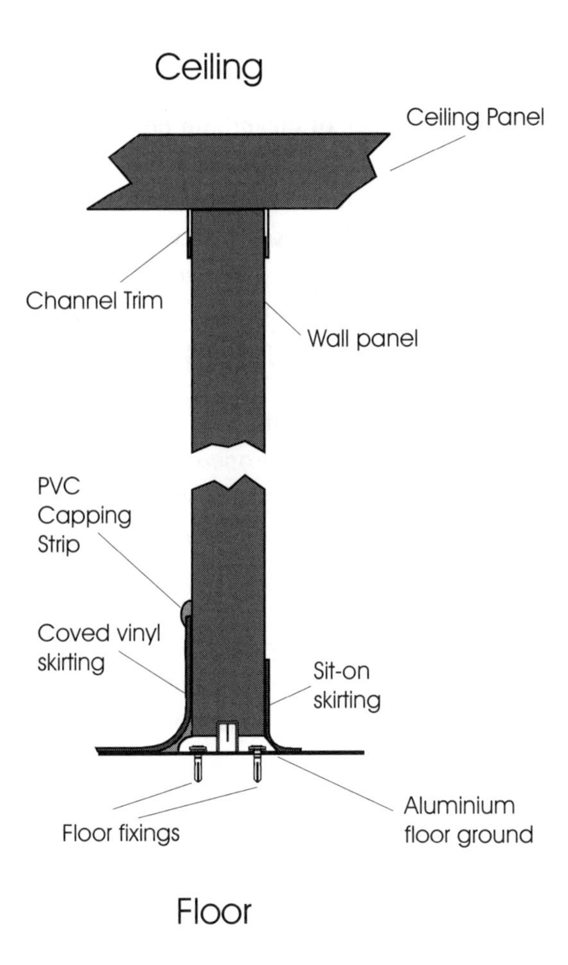

Figure 7.3 Cross-section of less expensive ceiling and floor details used in a modular construction system

Framed systems are also used where process machinery is isolated from the rest of the room. Isolators or minienvironments, as well as safety screens round machinery, are examples of this use. Lightweight aluminium extrusions are connected together to give a framework round the machinery and panels made of aluminium sheet, glass or clear plastic are glazed into the frames by use of special easy-to-clean gaskets.

7.4 Doors and Windows

Probably the most popular types of cleanroom doors are made either from plastic covered wood, or faced with mild steel that is suitably treated and painted. To assist cleaning and minimise hand contamination, door fittings such as door handles should be dispensed with where possible.

Doors would usually be hung so they would be kept closed by the positive pressure of the cleanroom. However, exceptions may be required so that personnel can pass through by pushing the door with their body. In that case, a self-closer should be fitted.

Doors are often manufactured with fine tolerances to minimise air leakage. This is a particularly useful property in a negatively pressurised containment room to minimise the entry of contamination from outside the room. However, in positively pressurised rooms this may be unnecessary, especially if the design requires air to flow through the doorway when open (see Section 5.1.4).

Doors may be glazed, which is particularly useful in the materials transfer airlock to see if it is occupied. If glazing is required, the method of glazing (i.e. gaskets) should allow easy cleaning. Doors that are completely made of glass are also available.

Windows are fitted to cleanrooms. These are useful in dissuading visitors who have come to see the cleanroom from entering; they are also necessary to allow management to see what is going on in the room without having the bother of changing into cleanroom clothing. Their number should, however be kept to a minimum. Windows should be glazed using easy-to-clean gaskets.

7.5 Floors

Concrete would be used as a common floor foundation in almost all cleanrooms. A smooth, impervious and durable surface would then be added. This should be resistant to spilled chemicals and be slip resistant. It may also be necessary in some situations to use materials that have good electrostatic or minimal outgassing properties.

A commonly used method of covering the floor is with vinyl sheeting that is welded together. A less common surface covering is terrazzo, which is very durable and is suitable in some situations.

Vinyl sheeting can be manufactured to be electrically conductive for use where this is desirable. In unidirectional flow rooms, where the air passes through the floor, it would be common to find that the floor is made of tiles placed on pedestals. If the room is used for semiconductor manufacturing, vinyl may not be an acceptable surface material because of the problem of 'outgassing'.

The floor-to-wall joints would normally be coved with some type of corner profile. An exception to this requirement may be where machines are used to clean the floor.

7.6 Ceilings

It would be unusual to have anything but a false ceiling in a cleanroom. The need for access to air conditioning ducts and other gas and electricity services, and the use of terminal filters and recessed lights that are integrated with the ceiling, dictates the use of a suspended or supported ceiling.

In conventionally ventilated cleanrooms the ceiling would be either of the suspended or self-supported type. Into the space between the support channels, the light fittings and air filter housings would be placed, the remaining areas being fitted with blank panels. Figure 7.4 is a photograph of a suspended cleanroom ceiling suitable for walking on, and showing the various components.

All of the light fittings, filter modules and blank panels must be well fitted to ensure a minimum of air leakage. If top-quality components are not used, mastic or other means can be used to bed down the various components.

In unidirectional flow cleanrooms, most of the ceiling is covered with filters. In that case, the ceiling is built of aluminium extruded channels and the filters are inserted into the channels. This is discussed in Sections 6.1.3 and 8.6 of this book.

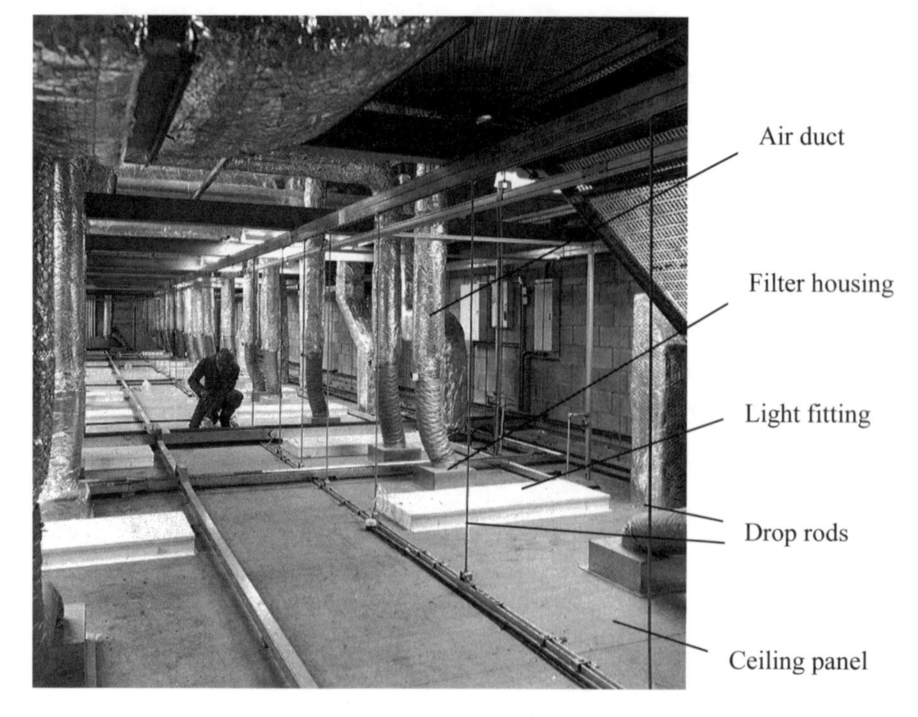

Figure 7.4 Suspended cleanroom ceiling

7.7 Outgassing and Electrostatic Properties

In semiconductor and similar areas, the use of construction materials that allow chemicals to 'outgas' can give contamination problems. Cleanroom flooring will often be plastic sheeting. Vinyl flooring is made of PVC with other materials added, one of these being a plasticiser to make it flexible. These plasticisers will outgas and are therefore not a good choice for semiconductor cleanrooms, especially as the floor has a large surface area. Some types of wall and ceiling panels may also be considered a risk. Another material that is considered a risk is silicon sealant used for sealing various joints. More suitable sealants can be purchased. Adhesives may also be a problem.

Test methods are available to ascertain the outgassing properties of materials. These can accelerate the 'outgassing' of contamination and assess the amount that will condense onto a surface.

If static charge is considered a problem, then the construction materials should be conductive and earthed to dissipate the electrostatic charge. However, if there is no electrical resistance there will be a danger to personnel through an electrical accident. It has been suggested that the electrical resistance should therefore be between 10^6 and 10^9 ohms/cm.

Acknowledgement

Figure 7.1 is reproduced with permission of Thermal Transfer. Figures 7.2, 7.3 and 7.4 are reproduced with permission of MSS Clean Technology.

8

High Efficiency Air Filtration

8.1 Air Filters used in Cleanrooms

The air supplied to a cleanroom must be filtered to ensure the removal of particles and micro-organisms. Until the early 1980s, High Efficiency Particulate Air (HEPA) filters filtered cleanroom air, as these were the most efficient air filters available. A HEPA filter has a minimum efficiency in removing small airborne particles, approximately equal to 0.3µm, of 99.97%. Today, HEPA filters are still used in most cleanrooms to remove the micro-organisms and inert particles in the supply air.

The production of integrated circuits has now evolved to a level where more efficient filters than HEPA filters are required to ensure that fewer and smaller particles pass through the air filters and into the cleanroom. Better filters are used and these are known as Ultra Low Penetration Air (ULPA) filters. An ULPA filter will have an efficiency greater than 99.999% against 0.1–0.2 µm particles. These filters are constructed and function in the same way as a HEPA filter.

It is generally accepted that

- For cleanrooms of ISO Class 6 (Class 1000) and poorer quality, HEPA filters are used with turbulent ventilation to meet the cleanroom classification.
- For ISO Class 5 (Class 100), HEPA filters that completely cover the ceiling are used to supply unidirectional flow down through the cleanroom.
- For ISO Class 4 (Class 10) or lower, ULPA filters should be used with unidirectional flow.

8.2 The Construction of High Efficiency Filters

High efficiency filters are usually constructed in two ways, i.e. deep-pleated or mini-pleated. In a deep-pleated filter, which is the more traditional construction method, rolls of filter paper are folded back and forward, side by side, either in 15 cm (6 inches) or 30 cm (12 inch) widths. To allow the air to pass through the paper and give the filter strength, a crinkled sheet of aluminium foil is often used as a separator. This pack of filter media and separators is then glued into a frame of a plastic, wood or metal. A cross-section of this traditional construction is shown in Figure 8.1.

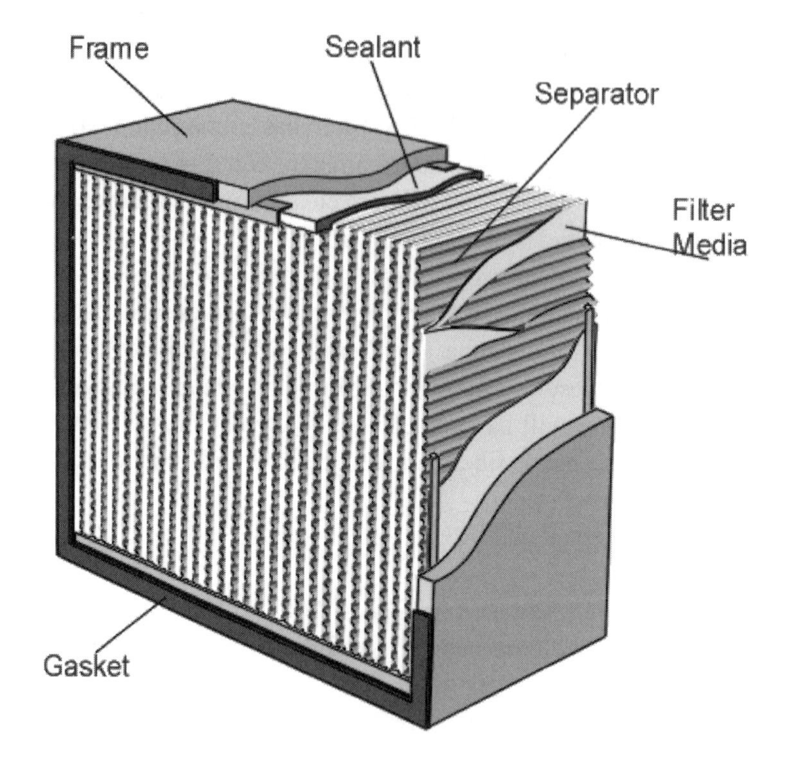

Figure 8.1 Deep-pleated high efficiency filter with separators

High efficiency filters are now most commonly available in a mini-pleat form. Aluminium separators are not used in this method of construction but the paper medium is folded over ribbons, glued strings, or raised dimples in the media and assembled into a frame. This method of assembly allows 2.5 to 3 times more pleats than the deep-pleated filters and can therefore be made more compact.

Mini-pleated construction is the most widely used method of construction for unidirectional flow cleanroom because the larger media area yields a lower pressure drop than deep-pleated construction. Such a method of construction is shown in Figure 8.2.

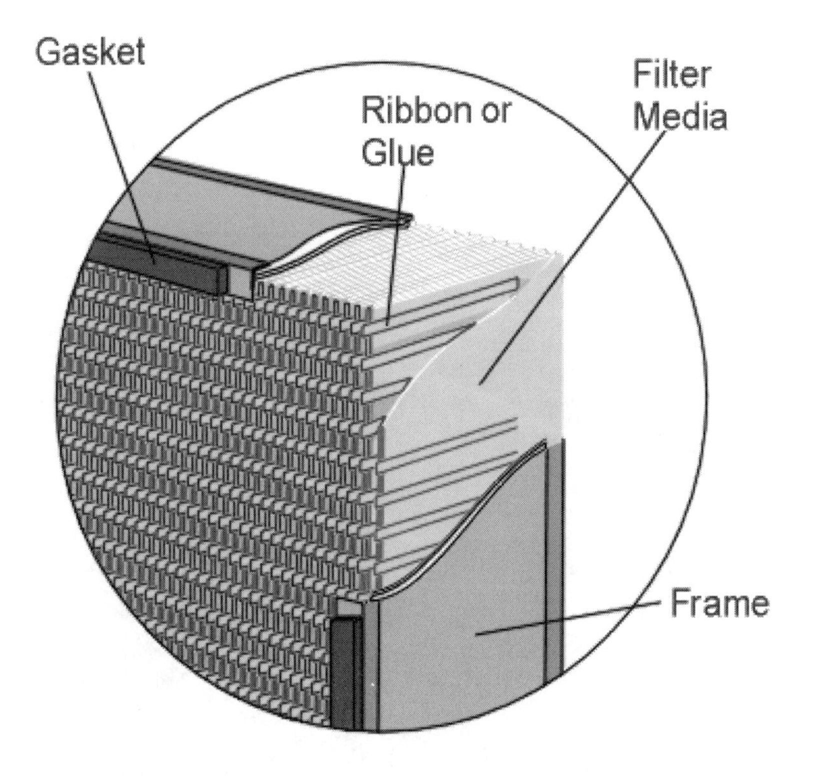

Figure 8.2 Section of a mini-pleated filter

The pressure drop across a filter is dependent on the air velocity through the filter media and its type of construction. The nominal air velocity through a filter is usually considered to be 0.5 m/s (100 ft/min). At this velocity the pressure drop is likely to be between 120 Pa and 170 Pa. When the pressure drop reaches 2.5 to 3 times the original pressure, the filters are normally replaced.

8.3 Particle Removal Mechanisms

A high efficiency filter is designed to remove particles of about 2 µm and smaller. Much less expensive pre-filters can be used to remove larger particles and these are not discussed in this chapter. High efficiency filter media is made of glass fibres ranging in diameter from as little as 0.1 µm and up to 10 µm, with spaces between fibres often very much larger than the particles captured. An ULPA filter will use a higher proportion of finer fibres than a HEPA filter.

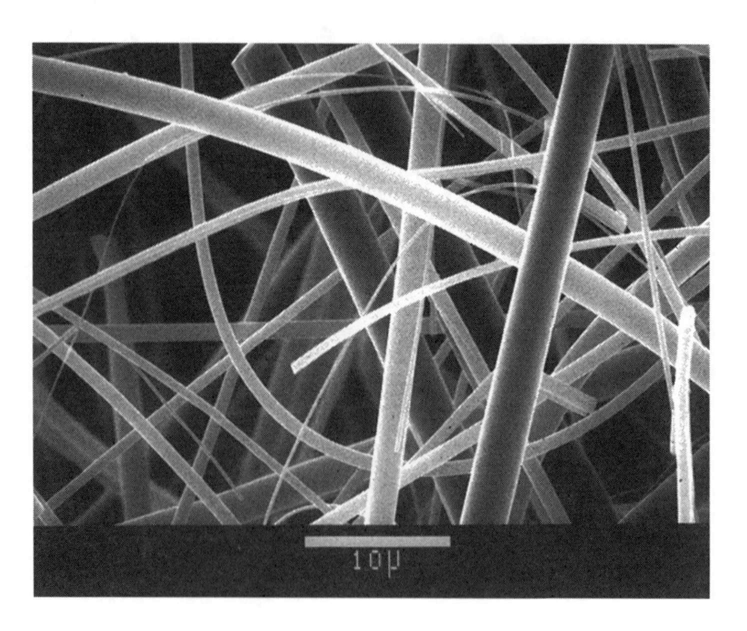

Figure 8.3 Photomicrograph of high efficiency filter media

These fibres criss-cross randomly throughout the depth of the filter media and do not give a controlled pore size. A photomicrograph of high efficiency filter media is shown in Figure 8.3. A 10 μm scale is shown at the base of the photograph.

As airborne particles move through the filter paper, they bump into the fibres, or onto other particles that are already stuck to the fibres. When a particle bumps into either a fibre or a particle, strong forces, such as Van der Waal's, are established between the captured particle and the fibre or particle that has captured it; these retain the particle.

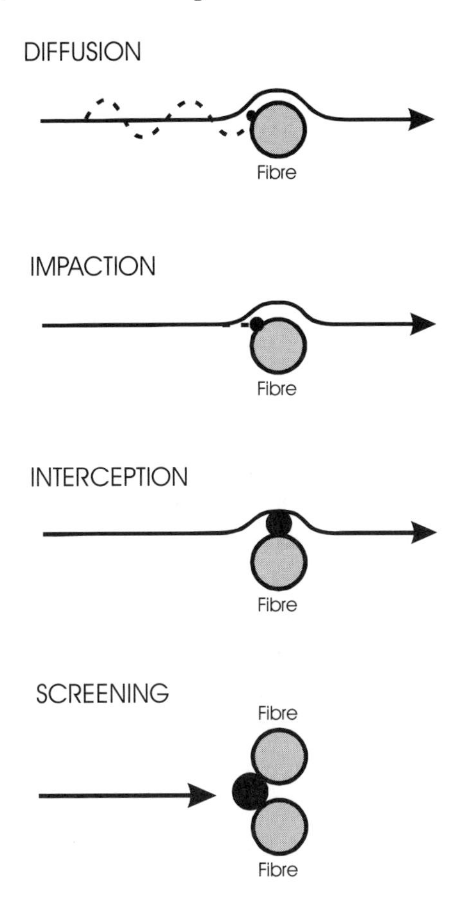

Figure 8.4 Particle removal mechanisms

The three main mechanisms involved in the removal of small particles in filter media are impaction, diffusion and interception. Sieving or straining is of much less importance as this occurs only with larger particles sizes that are removed by primary filters placed before the high efficiency filters. These four mechanisms are shown diagrammatically in Figure 8.4. It may be assumed that electrostatic effects are generally unimportant in high efficiency filters and for that reason are not included in the figure.

In the process of capture by *diffusion* (also known as Brownian movement), small particles (i.e. those without sufficient mass to leave the gas stream on their own) move about randomly. This random motion from these small particles is caused by constant bombardment by other small particles and the molecules of the gas in which they are suspended. This random motion causes the smaller particles to move about and they may touch the fibres of the filter or previously captured particles.

In the process of capture by *impaction*, particles large enough (i.e. with enough mass) to have sufficient momentum leave the gas stream and strike a fibre as the gas turns around a fibre. If a particle strikes a fibre as it passes it, i.e. tangentially, it will be captured and retained, this mechanism being known as *interception*. The final mechanism of filtration, which is known as *sieving* or straining, occurs when the spaces between the fibres are smaller than the particles that are being captured.

A high efficiency filter is dependent on the first three of the mechanisms described above to remove particles in the air. The largest size of particles is removed by inertial impaction, the medium size by direct interception and the smallest by diffusion. This concept is demonstrated in Figure 8.5. This figure shows the classical removal efficiency curve for a HEPA-type filter and a minimum efficiency for a particle size of about 0.3 μm. This 'most penetrating size' normally varies between 0.1 μm and 0.3 μm. It also is interesting to note that high efficiency filters are more efficient against particles than are smaller than the most penetrating size; this effect is caused by diffusion.

The curve gives a rather simplistic approach. It is known that the particle size that has the minimum removal efficiency (or the maximum penetrating particle size) varies depending on variables such as the density of a particle and the type of filter medium.

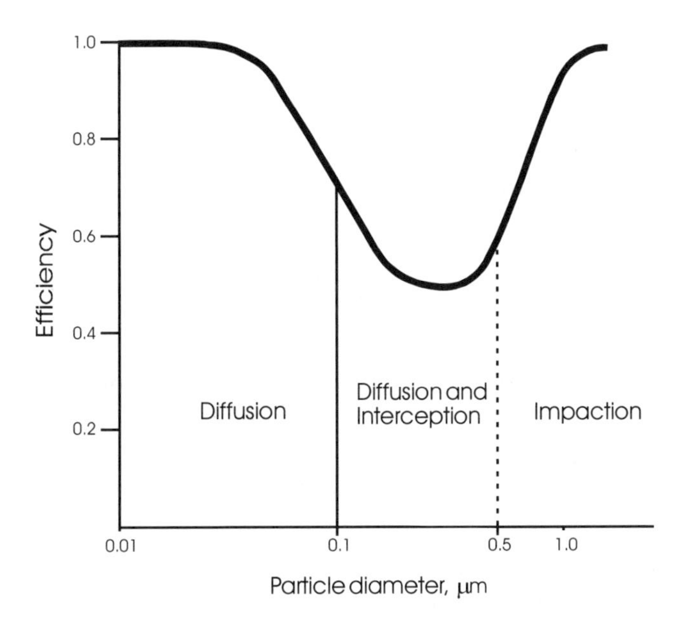

Figure 8.5 Classical efficiency curve for an air filter

8.4 Testing of High Efficiency Filters

High efficiency filters are tested after manufacture to measure their efficiency against test particles. There are a number of tests used for this purpose. The best known are:

8.4.1 Military Standard 282

This USA test originally used thermally generated particles of di-octyl phthalate (DOP) with an average size of 0.3 μm to test the efficiency of HEPA filters. However, other oils such as poly-alpha olefin (PAO) or di-octyl sebacate (DOS) have replaced DOP. Heating such an oil produces an oil mist, and the efficiency against this challenge is determined.

8.4.2 Sodium Flame Test (Eurovent 4/4)

This European test method for HEPA filters uses an aerosol of particles of sodium chloride that have a mass median size of 0.6 μm. The test aerosol is sprayed into the air as an aqueous solution and the dry particles that are formed are used to determine the filter's efficiency.

8.4.3 Institute of Environmental Sciences (IEST) Recommended Practice 'Testing ULPA Filters'.

The Institute of Environmental Sciences and Technology (IEST) has developed a Recommended Practice for testing ULPA filters (IEST-RP-CC007). An optical particle counter is used to measure particles, although a condensation nuclei counter can be used to extend the lower range. The choice of the aerosol material is left to the user, but must meet certain optical properties. This test system provides a particle size efficiency in size ranges from around 0.07 μm to 3.0 μm.

8.4.4 European Standard (EN 1822)

This standard is used for both HEPA and ULPA filters and gives a method for testing the particle removal efficiency and classifying the filter.

An important departure of this test method from the methods outlined above is the determination of the Most Penetrating Particle Size (MPPS) for the filter media being tested, and the measurement of the removal efficiency of the filter at that particle size. As discussed in Section 8.3, each filter has a particular particle size that will pass through the filter most easily, that size being determined by variables, such as the fibre content of the filter media, air velocity and its packing density. It is logical therefore to test the filter at that most penetrating particle size. The MPPS is normally between 0.1 μm and 0.3 μm.

The first stage of this test method is to determine the MPPS of the flat sheet filter medium used in the filter. This is carried out at the face velocity that will correspond with that produced by the filter when working at its given flow rates. The efficiency of the complete filter can then be determined in two ways:

- Leak testing (local efficiency). The filter media of the complete filter is scanned to determine the amount of leakage through pinholes in the filter medium.
- Overall efficiency. The efficiency of the complete filter is determined at its rated flow.

The filter is then classified by its overall and local efficiency against its most penetrating particle. This classification is shown in Table 8.1.

Table 8.1 Classification of filters according to the EN 1822.

Filter class	Overall value efficiency (%)	Overall value penetration (%)	Leak test Efficiency (%)	Leak test penetration (%)
H 10	85	15	–	–
H 11	95	5	–	–
H 12	99.5	0.5	–	–
H 13	99.95	0.05	99.75	0.25
H 14	99.995	0.005	99.975	0.025
U 15	99.999 5	0.000 5	99.997 5	0.002 5
U 16	99.999 95	0.000 05	99.999 75	0.000 25
U 17	99.999 995	0.000 005	99.999 9	0.000 1

8.5 Probe (Scan) Testing of High Efficiency Filters

Air that is supplied in a turbulently ventilated cleanroom through diffusers in the ceiling is thoroughly mixed with the room air. Some pinhole leaks in the filters can be tolerated, as long as they are not great enough to significantly reduce the overall efficiency of the filtration system and affect the required air cleanliness. This tolerance is possible because the small number of particles passing through the filter are well mixed with the room air.

This is not the case in unidirectional flow systems, where a leak can release a unidirectional stream of particles into the close proximity of the process or product. To prevent these pinhole leaks, the filters should be scanned in the factory by introducing a test dust before the filter and scanning the whole filter with overlapping passes using a probe and searching for leaks. This method is very similar to that described in Chapter 12 of this book.

8.6 Filter Housings for High Efficiency Filters

When a high efficiency filter leaves the factory where it has been manufactured and tested, it should be fit for the purpose required. If it has been properly packed and transported, and installed by personnel who are familiar with the delicate nature of filter media, then the filter's integrity should be maintained.

To ensure that there is no ingress of unfiltered air into the cleanroom, the filter must be fitted into a well-designed housing. The housing must be of sound construction and particular attention must be paid to the method of housing/filter sealing.

Neoprene rubber gaskets are commonly fitted to the filter frame as seals. This is illustrated in Figure 8.1. When the filter is fitted into the filter housing the gasket presses down, compressing onto a flat face of the housing and preventing the leakage of contaminated air (Figure 8.6). This method is normally successful, but distortion of the filter frame or housings, as supplied or when tightening up, as well as poor or old gaskets, can cause leakage. Better-designed housings overcome these problems.

Figure 8.7 shows a system that would be used in a unidirectional flow cleanroom. The ceiling grid has a continuous channel filled with the fluid seal, which is a jelly-like substance that will not flow out of the channel. A knife-edge fitted to the filter frame mates into the channel of sealant. The fluid flows round the knife-edge to give a perfect seal and prevents particles by-passing the filter through the housing.

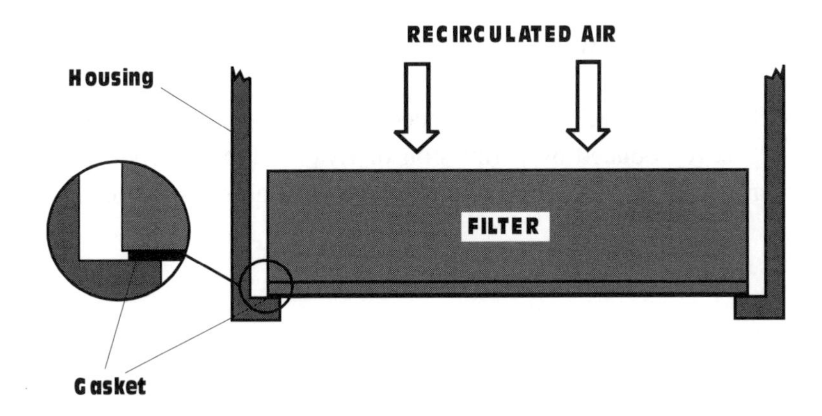

Figure 8.6 Traditional neoprene gasket sealing method

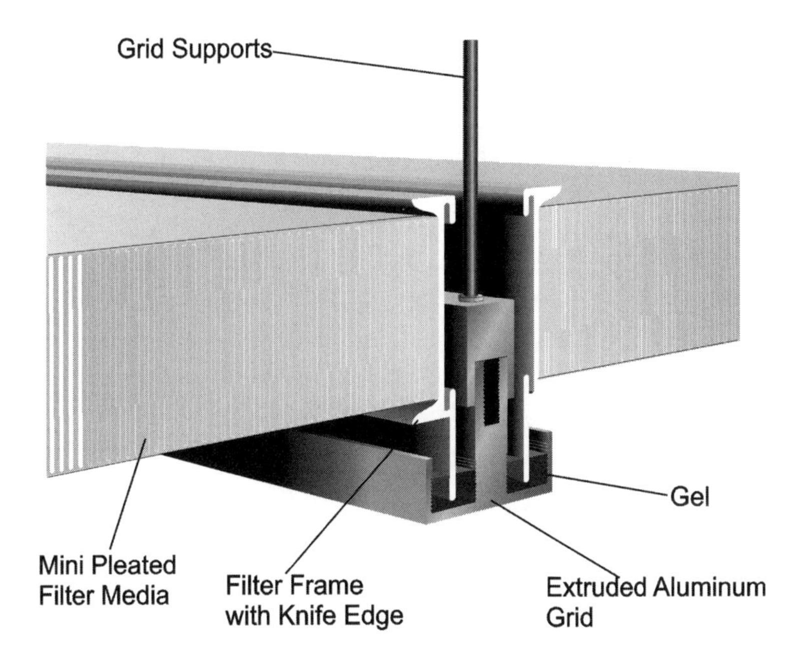

Figure 8.7 Ceiling grid with channel for a fluid seal

Acknowledgements

Figures 8.1, 8.2 and 8.7 are reproduced by permission of Flanders Filters. Figure 8.3 is reproduced by permission of Evanite Fiber Corporation. Table 8.1 is reproduced by permission of the British Standards Institution.

9

Cleanroom Testing and Monitoring

When a cleanroom has been built and about to be handed over to the purchaser, or when an existing cleanroom is reopened after being shut down for modifications that could cause changes to its contamination control characteristics, it will be tested. This initial type of testing is to establish that the cleanroom is working correctly and achieving the contamination standards that it has been designed to fulfil. These standards are laid down in ISO 14644-1. A secondary function of this initial testing is to establish the initial performance of the room so that this can be adopted as a 'benchmark'. When the room is checked in the future, either routinely or when a contamination problem is encountered, deviations from the original conditions may be found, and the possible reasons for contamination thus ascertained. The final and indirect reason for carrying out initial testing of a cleanroom is to familiarise and train the staff who will monitor and run the room. This may be their most important, and possibly only, opportunity to understand how their cleanroom works and learn the methods used to test and ensure that the cleanroom continues to perform correctly.

When it has been shown that the cleanroom fulfils the ISO 14664-1 cleanroom classification set down at the design stage, it is necessary to regularly check the room at the time intervals set by ISO 14644-2, to ensure that the room continues to comply with the standard. Many cleanrooms are built and passed over to the user with little or no effort being put into ensuring that over its many years of use the correct level of cleanliness continues to be achieved. Testing must therefore be carried out so that the customer who buys the product made within the room gets a product that is fit for the purpose it is intended.

As well as checking the cleanroom to show that it is working correctly when first installed and at regular intervals to show that it complies with ISO 14644-1, it may be necessary to regularly monitor the room. This may not be required in poorer cleanrooms, but in higher quality rooms it may be necessary to monitor the room to ensure that the correct conditions are maintained during production. This testing may be either continually, or at intervals that are much shorter that those laid down in ISO 14644-2 to show continued complience.

Most of the tests carried out to test the initial performance, or demonstrate continual compliance, are identical to those used to monitor it, although it is normal to find that the initial testing is more thorough and extensive.

9.1. Principles of Cleanroom Testing

To show that a cleanroom is working satisfactorily it is necessary to demonstrate that the following principles have been satisfied:

- The air supplied to the cleanroom is of sufficient *quantity* to dilute or remove the contamination generated in the room.
- The air within the cleanroom suite moves from clean to less-clean areas to minimise the movement of contaminated air. Air should move in the correct direction through doorways and the fabric of the room.
- The air supplied to the cleanroom is of a *quality* that will not add significantly to the contamination within the room.
- The air movement within the cleanroom should ensure that there are no areas within the room with high concentrations of contamination

If these principles are satisfied then the concentration of particles, and where necessary microbe-carrying particles, should be measured to ascertain that the specified cleanroom standard has been achieved.

9.2 Cleanroom Tests

To ensure that the requirements in Section 9.1 are fulfilled, the tests shown in Figure 9.1 should be carried out, preferably in the order given.

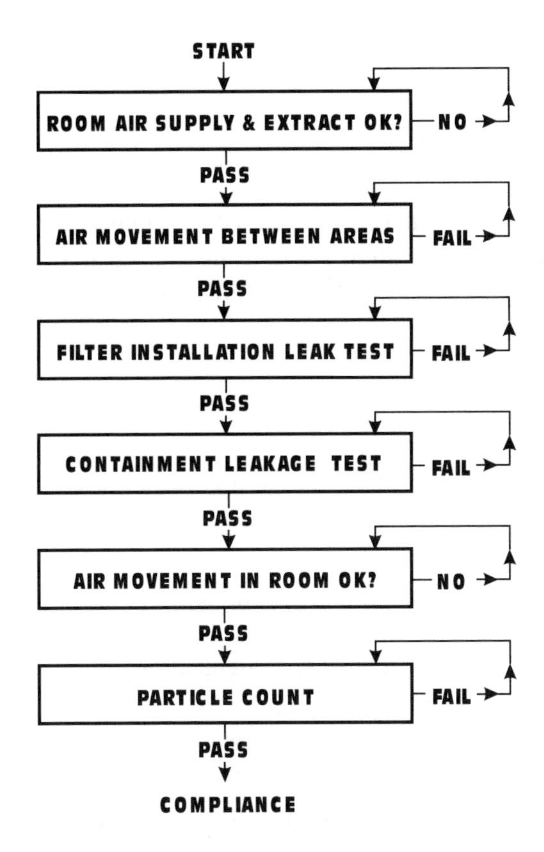

Figure 9.1 Cleanroom test sequence

9.2.1 Air supply and extract quantities

In the case of turbulently ventilated cleanrooms the air supply and extract volumes should be measured. In the case of unidirectional airflow it should be the air velocity.

9.2.2 Air movement control between areas

To demonstrate that the airflow between areas is in the correct direction i.e. from the clean to the less-clean, it is necessary to check that:

- The pressure differences between areas are correct.
- The air direction through doorways, hatches, etc. is from clean to less-clean.

9.2.3 Filter installation leak test

The high efficiency air filter, and its housing, should be checked to ensure that no airborne contamination passes into the cleanroom through (a) a damaged filter (b) between the filter and its housing or (c) any other part of the filter installation.

9.2.4 Containment leak testing

Testing should be carried out to show that airborne contamination is not entering the cleanroom through its construction materials.

9.2.5 Air movement control within the room

The type of air movement control tests depend on whether the room is turbulently or unidirectionally ventilated. If the cleanroom is turbulently ventilated then it is necessary to check that there are no areas within the room with insufficient air movement. If the room has unidirectional airflow, it is necessary to check that the air velocity and direction throughout the room is that specified in the design.

9.2.6 Airborne particles and microbial concentrations

If the above tests are satisfactory then final measurements will be carried out to ascertain that the concentration of particles, and where appropriate micro-organisms, comply with the design specification laid down for the room.

9.2.7 Additional tests

As well as these contamination control tests, it may be necessary to satisfy one or more of the following requirements:

- temperature
- relative humidity
- heating and cooling capabilities of the room
- sound levels
- lighting levels
- vibration levels.

These additional requirements are not considered in any detail in this book, as they are tests that may be required in air conditioned rooms other than cleanrooms. Information on these types of tests are available in various building services textbooks and in Guides provided by the American Society Heating Refrigeration and Airconditioning Engineers (ASHRAE) in the USA, and the Chartered Institute of Building Services Engineers (CIBSE) in the UK.

9.3 Testing in Relation to Room Type and Occupation State

The type of tests to be carried out in a cleanroom depend on whether the room is unidirectional, turbulent or mixed airflow (a mixed flow room is one that is turbulently ventilated but has unidirectional flow cabinets, workstations, or isolators within the room). The types of tests required with respect to the type of cleanroom are discussed in the chapters that follow.

Tests can be carried out in the cleanroom when it is (a) 'as-built' i.e. in the empty room, (b) 'at rest' i.e. the room fitted with machinery but no personnel present or (c) 'fully operational'. These occupancy states are discussed more fully in Section 3.4 of this book. When the cleanroom is being handed over to the user the initial testing is usually done in the 'as built' condition. Similarly, when the cleanroom is checked throughout its life to demonstrate that it complies with ISO 14644-1, it will be normally tested in the 'at rest' condition. This will demonstrate that the cleanroom is working correctly. However, if the cleanroom is being monitored to demonstrate that the conditions in the room are acceptable for production, the testing will be done in the 'fully operational' condition. The type of tests required in each of the occupational states are very similar and any differences are described in next few chapters.

9.4 Re-testing to Demonstrate Compliance

It is necessary to ensure that a cleanroom performs satisfactorily throughout its life and continues to comply with its cleanroom classification. The cleanroom must therefore be checked at regular intervals, these intervals being more frequent in higher specified rooms.

Table 9.2 Schedule of tests to demonstrate continuing compliance.

Test Parameter	Class	Maximum Time Interval
To demonstrate compliance by particle counting	≤ ISO 5	6 months
	> ISO 5	12 months
Schedule of additional tests		
Airflow velocity or volume	all classes	12 months
Air pressure difference	all classes	12 months
Schedule of optional tests		
Installed filter leakage	all classes	24 months*
Airflow visualisation	all classes	24 months*
Recovery	all classes	24 months*
Containment leakage	all classes	24 months*

*= suggested time interval

ISO 14644-2 gives the maximum time interval that a cleanroom should be left before being tested to show it still complies with ISO 14644-1. These maximum time intervals are listed in Table 9.2 along with the type of test. The one test that must be carried out to demonstrate that a cleanroom continues to comply with ISO 14644-1 is particle concentration testing. This must be carried out at a maximum time interval of 6 months for a cleanroom with a classification of ≤ ISO Class 5, or 12 months if the classification is over ISO Class 5. Particle counting tests are normally carried out in the 'at-rest' state but may also be carried out in the 'operational' state. If the installation has a continuous, or frequent, particle and air pressure difference monitoring system, then ISO 14644-2 allows the time interval to be extended.

Where the application requires them, 'additional' tests to demonstrate compliance are added. These are air velocity or volume, and air pressure difference testing. These must be tested at a maximum interval of 12 months, although the time interval can be extended if continuous, or frequent, monitoring is used.

The ISO 14644-2 standard also allow 'optional' tests to be included in the testing if agreed by customer and supplier. These should be tested at a maximum test interval of 24 months. However, in this case these are only suggested time intervals. These tests are as follows:

- The filter is installed correctly.
- The air movement within the cleanroom is correct i.e. airflow visualization tests.
- Any contamination dispersed is removed efficiently i.e. recovery test.
- The air is moving in the correct direction through the cleanroom fabric, i.e. from clean to less-clean.

All of the above tests are discussed in subsequent chapters of this book.

9.5 Monitoring of Cleanrooms

The time intervals, and tests to be carried out, to show that a cleanroom continues to comply with ISO standard 14644-1 are provided in ISO

14644-2. In cleanrooms of a high standard, where cleanliness is a vital part of the production process, further testing or monitoring, may be required. This will be carried out to show that during production the cleanroom conditions are acceptable, and under control. It is suggested in ISO 14644-2 that the user should use a risk assessment to decide what monitoring tests should be done and how often.

The variables that are most likely to be monitored are:

- air pressure difference
- airborne particle count
- where appropriate, microbiological counts.

Air pressure difference can be measured and recorded continuously by measuring instruments. This might be necessary in high quality cleanrooms such as ISO Class 4, and better. If monitoring is done in cleanrooms of poorer quality, the time interval might be daily, weekly, monthly, three monthly or six monthly intervals, the interval being shorter as cleanroom classification becomes cleaner. Some further information is given in Chapter 15.

Particle counts can be measured and recorded using the same criterion discussed in the previous paragraph. It should be noted that when particle counts are monitored, it is not expected that this should be done at the number or layout of positions laid down in ISO 14644-1. Much fewer positions can be selected and they need not be distributed evenly around the cleanroom. Monitoring positions should be selected that are important to production e.g. close to where the product is exposed to contamination.

Acknowledgements

Table 9.2 is compiled from information given in ISO 14644-2 and reproduced by permission of the British Standards Institution.

10

Measurement of Air Quantities and Pressure Differences

A cleanroom must have sufficient clean air supplied to dilute and remove the airborne contamination generated within the room. In a turbulently ventilated cleanroom its cleanliness classification is directly related to the air supply; the more air supplied in a given time, the cleaner the room. In a unidirectional cleanroom, the cleanroom classification is dependent on the air supply velocity. These volumes and velocities will have been decided at the design stage. It will therefore be necessary at the initial testing of the design, and at regular intervals throughout the cleanroom's life, to measure and show that the air quantities are correct.

To ensure that the air in a cleanroom always moves from clean to less-clean areas, a positive pressure difference between the areas will have to be set up. This is normally done when the correct air supply and extract volumes are set up, i.e. the air conditioning plant is balanced. This is discussed in Section 5.1.4 of this book.

10.1 Air Quantities

Specialist firms usually carry out the measurement and adjustment of the air supply and extract volumes when the cleanroom is commissioned. However, simple tests can be used to verify that these air flow quantities continue to be maintained. Several types of instruments can be used to measure air quantities. Those commonly used in cleanrooms fall into the following groups:

- hoods for measuring air supply volumes;
- anemometers for measuring air velocities.

In turbulently ventilated rooms, the supply and extract air volumes can be measured within the air conditioning ducts. Specialist firms using instruments such as a Pitot-static tube normally do this.

The Pitot-static tube is inserted into the air duct and used to measure the velocities across the duct; the air supply volumes can then be calculated. However, it is also common to measure these air volumes from within the cleanroom.

10.1.1 Measuring air quantities from within a cleanroom

If the room air is supplied through a terminal air filter, without an air diffuser, then the air supply can be determined by use of an anemometer at the filter face. If the average velocity is found, then the air volume is calculated by multiplying that velocity by the area of the filter. However, because of the non-uniformity of the air velocity across the filter and at the edge of the filter, the average velocity is difficult to determine; it is therefore difficult to accurately measure the air supply volume.

When air supply diffusers are used, the unevenness of the throw of air from around the diffusers, and hence the air velocities, make it almost impossible to measure the correct air volume. Similar problems occur at extract grilles, but the air velocity is more even and the use of an anemometer will give reasonable readings.

It is best to use a hood similar to the type shown in the Figure 10.1 to measure the air supply volumes. The hood is lifted up to the ceiling and encloses the air supply diffuser. The supply air is then gathered together and an average velocity, and hence the volume per unit time, measured at the exit of the hood. This method overcomes the problems discussed in the previous two paragraphs.

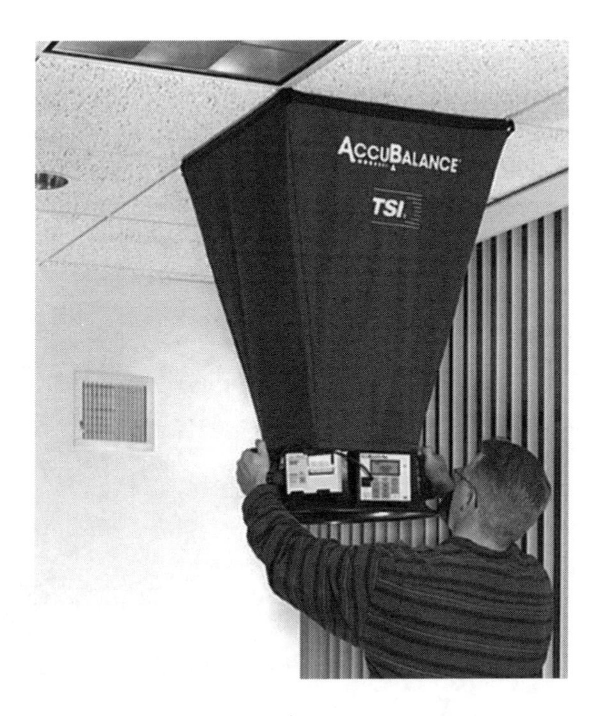

Figure 10.1 Flow measuring hood

10.1.2 Anemometers

Anemometers are used to measure the velocity of the air being supplied from a high efficiency filter used in unidirectional flow. The anemometer has to be far enough away from the filter to allow the unevenness of the air coming from the filter to become more uniform. A distance of about 30cm (12 inches) from the filter is about correct.

10.1.2.1 Vane anemometer

These instruments measure velocity and work on the principle of air turning a vane, each turn usually being measured electronically and the frequency of impulses converted into a velocity.

An example of a vane anemometer is shown in Figure 10.2. If the velocity to be measured is less than about 0.2 m/s (40 ft/min), the mechanical friction in some anemometers may affect the turning of the vane.

Some vane anemometers can average the velocity over an extended time interval. This is a useful attribute, as the velocity of air from filters, and within the cleanroom space, fluctuates quite a bit. It can therefore be difficult to obtain a correct average reading without such a facility.

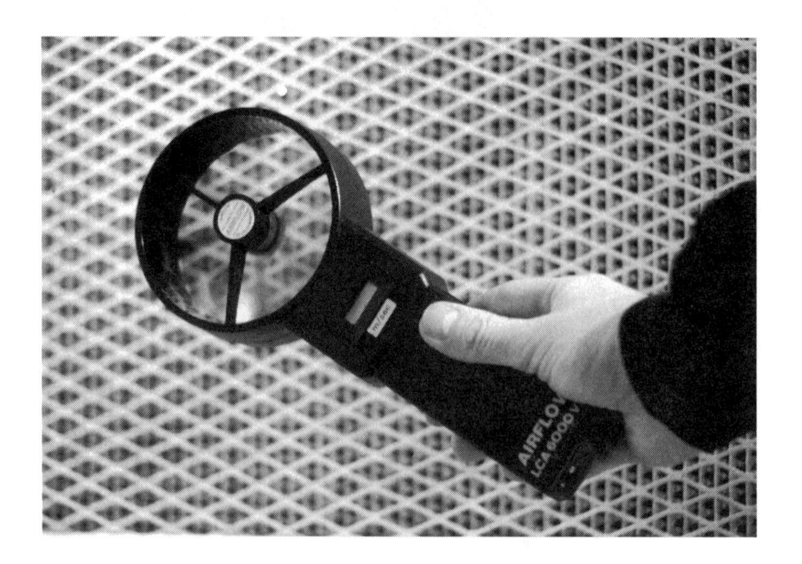

Figure 10.2 Vane anemometer

10.1.2.2 Thermal anemometers

This type of anemometer uses the cooling effect of air passing through the head of the instrument to determine the air velocity. Different types exist, but a common type uses a bead thermistor, it's cooling being in proportion to the velocity. An example of this type of instrument is shown in Figure 10.3.

Low velocities can be measured with this type of apparatus and they are therefore suitable for use within cleanrooms. However, because of the air velocity fluctuations, average readings can be difficult to obtain accurately.

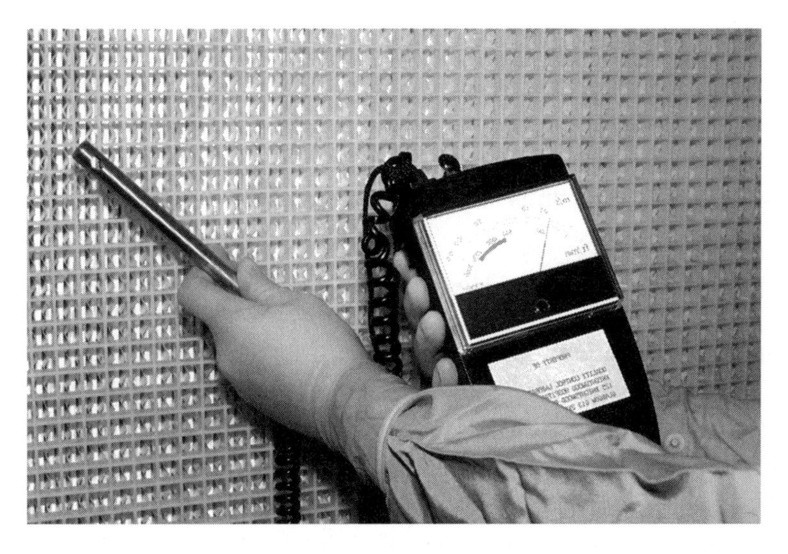

Figure 10.3 Thermal Anemometer

10.2 Differential Pressure Tests

It is necessary to ensure that air moves in a cleanroom suite from a clean to a less-clean area, and not vice-versa. Measurement of pressure is an indirect measurement of this, as air will flow from an area of high pressure to an area of lower pressure. The higher quality cleanrooms should therefore have a higher pressure than adjacent less-clean areas. The units of measurement used to register pressure differences are Pascals, although older units such as inch water gauge are sometimes used (12Pa = 0.05 inch water gauge). A pressure difference of 10 or 15 Pa is generally accepted as that which should be established between clean areas. 15 Pa is commonly used between a cleanroom and an unclassified room, and 10 Pa between two cleanrooms.

Problems can occur when trying to achieve a pressure difference between areas connected by large openings, such as a supply tunnel. To achieve the suggested pressure drop it may be necessary to use very large air quantities through the tunnel, even where the area of the opening has been restricted, or to accept a lower pressure difference. To accept a lower pressure difference is perfectly reasonable as long as the primary requirement is achieved, i.e. the airflow is always in the correct direction. It may, however, be difficult to convince everyone of the correctness of this argument, and it may be necessary to conform to cleanroom standards, which are normally stated in terms of pressure difference.

10.2.1 Apparatus for measuring pressure differences

A manometer capable of reading pressure differences in the range of 0–60 Pa (0–0.25 inch water) is required for measuring the pressure difference between rooms. This is usually an inclined manometer, magnehelic gauge, or electronic manometer.

The inclined manometer works by pressure pushing a liquid up an inclined tube. The inclined gauge shown in Figure 10.4 measures small pressure changes in the inclined tube up to a pressure of about 60 Pa. After that pressure, the tube moves round to the vertical where the distance that the column of liquid moves, for a given pressure, becomes smaller. This then allows larger pressure difference to be measured and this type of gauge can also be used for applications, such as measuring a pressure drop over an air filter, where the pressure differences can be in the 100 to 500 Pa range.

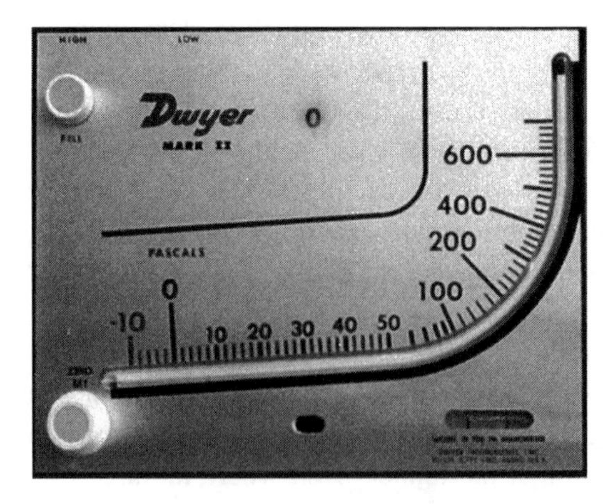

Figure 10.4 Inclined manometer

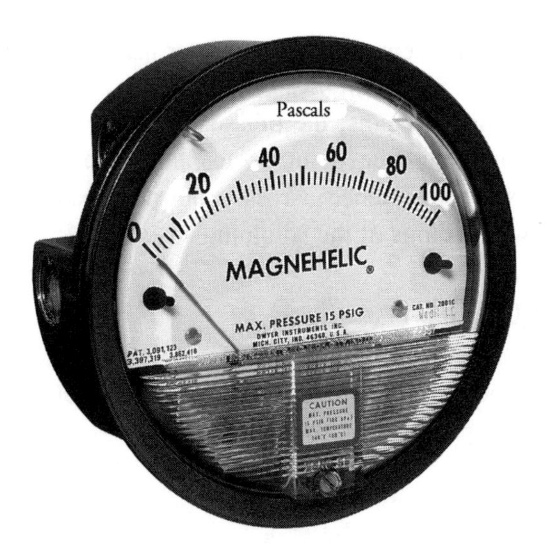

Figure 10.5 Magnehelic pressure gauge

The magnehelic gauge shown in Figure 10.5 works by the pressure acting on a diaphragm. This moves an indicating pointer, the movement being relayed through a magnetic linkage.

A series of manometers are often mounted on the outside of the cleanroom so that the pressure differences can be easily seen and checked. Pressures can also be relayed electronically from manometers to a room management system.

10.2.2 Methods of checking pressure differences

To check the pressure differences between areas, the air conditioning plant must be supplying and extracting the correct volumes of air and all doors in the cleanroom suite must be closed. If the pressure difference needs adjusting the air extract from the room must be reduced to increase the pressure, and opened to decrease it.

If manometers are not permanently installed, a tube from a pressure gauge is passed under the door, or through an open by-pass grille or damper into the adjacent area. It must be well clear of the door so that no pressure is registered from air movement along the floor near the door. A reading of the pressure difference may then be taken.

In some ventilation systems, the pressures within rooms are measured with respect to one reference point. When this type of system is being checked, the pressure difference across a doorway can be calculated by subtracting the two readings of the adjoining spaces.

Acknowledgements

Figure 10.1 is reproduced by permission of TSI Inc. Figures 10.4 and 10.5 are reproduced by permission of Dwyer Ltd.

11

Air Movement Control Between and Within Cleanrooms

11.1 Cleanroom Containment Leak Testing

To show that a cleanroom is working correctly, it is necessary to demonstrate that no contamination infiltrates into the cleanroom from dirtier adjacent areas. Airborne contamination can come from areas adjacent to the cleanroom through doors and hatches, as well as through holes and cracks in the walls, ceilings and other parts of the cleanroom fabric. If a cleanroom is pressurised correctly with respect to all adjacent areas, then air will flow out to areas of lower pressure and contamination will not enter the cleanroom. However, it is possible that adjacent areas such as air plenums or service ducts are at a higher pressure than the cleanroom and this may be overlooked.

An example of such a problem is shown is Figure 11.1. It can be seen in this drawing that a supply air plenum of a vertical unidirectional flow system is at a higher pressure than the cleanroom. Contamination can then be pushed into the cleanroom at the (a) ceiling-to-wall interface, (b) filter and lighting housings-to-ceiling interfaces, (c) ceiling-to-column interface, and (d) through the cladding of the ceiling support pillars.

Other infiltration problems are associated with service plenums and the entry of services into the cleanroom. For example, electrical sockets and switches, and other types of services providers, can be linked by conduits and ducts to dirty areas that are at a higher pressure than the cleanroom.

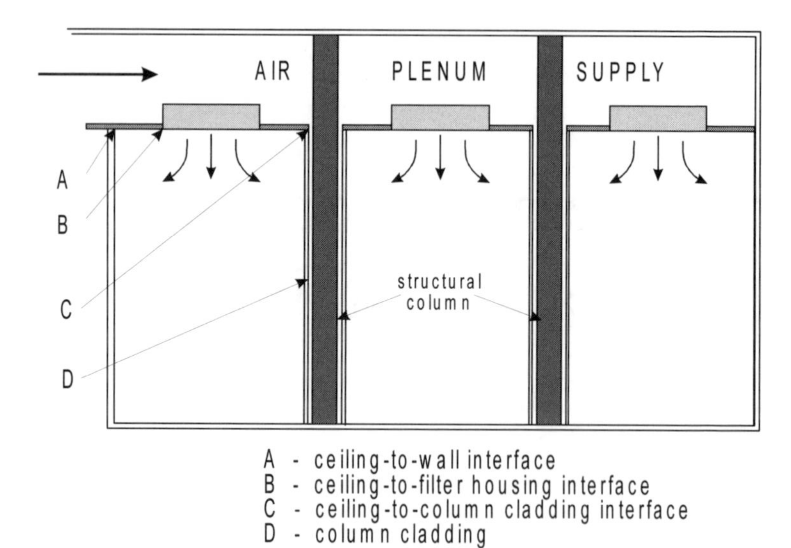

Figure 11.1 Infiltration problems with an air supply plenum

These problems are particularly difficult to foresee and control in a negatively pressurised containment room.

11.1.1 Methods of checking infiltration

It is a relatively simple matter to check that air is flowing in the correct direction through an open door, or through the cracks around a closed door. Generating smoke and observing air movement does this. However, to ensure that there is no unwanted flow of airborne contamination into a cleanroom through cracks at the walls, ceiling, floor and filter housings, etc., it is necessary to check these cracks. This will normally be at the overlapping edges or butted joints, as well as any other places where the cleanroom fabric is penetrated by, for example, service ducts or conduits.

A test dust or smoke can be introduced into the areas where the containment arises and possible areas of penetration scanned with a particle counter. This is not an easy task. Where the containment originates from may be unknown, and it is often difficult to find the places to release test smoke. In these cases, it should be sufficient to scan for particles, relying on the natural contamination that comes from the adjacent contaminated areas to show up any problem; if no particles show up in these circumstances the problem is unlikely to be serious.

Containment leak testing should be done in the cleanroom prior to handing it over to the user, or when major reconstruction work has been carried out. The ISO cleanroom standard 14644-2 lists the 'containment leak' test as an 'optional' test and suggest a re-testing interval of two years (see Table 9.2).

11.2 Air Movement Control within a Cleanroom

As part of the testing procedure to ensure that a cleanroom is working correctly, the air movement within the room should be checked. It is necessary to check that there is sufficient air movement within the room to either dilute, or remove, airborne contamination and hence prevent a build-up of contamination.

In a turbulently ventilated cleanroom, air is supplied and mixed in a turbulent way. Good mixing should be demonstrated in all parts of this type of cleanroom to ensure that contaminants will be removed. However, it is particularly important in critical areas, where the product is exposed to the risk of contamination, to demonstrate that good mixing is obtained.

In a unidirectional flow, to ensure the cleanest conditions, critical areas should be supplied with air coming directly from the high efficiency filters. However, problems may be encountered because of:

- heat rising from the machinery and disrupting the airflow;
- obstructions preventing the supply air getting to the critical area;
- obstructions, or the machinery shape, turning the unidirectional flow into turbulent flow;
- contamination being entrained into the clean air.

Visualising the airflow will demonstrate whether or not any of these problems exist and whether they are likely to cause an increase in contamination.

11.2.1 Air movement visualisation

There are a number of methods that can be used to visualise the flow of the air in a cleanroom. These can be grouped under the following headings:

1. streamers
2. smoke or particle streams
3. air velocity and direction measurement.

11.2.1.1 Streamers

The types of streamers that are used to visualise airflow are threads or tapes. The best type are those which have a high surface-area-to-weight ratio, and can be easily seen. Recording tapes of the type used in music cassettes can be used, as can loosely spun threads. A useful way of using streamers is to attach it onto the end of an anemometer; it can then be used to ascertain the direction of air when the velocity is being measured at a particular spot. Streamers can also be used by attaching a number of them onto a grid similar to that discussed in the Section 11.2.1.3.

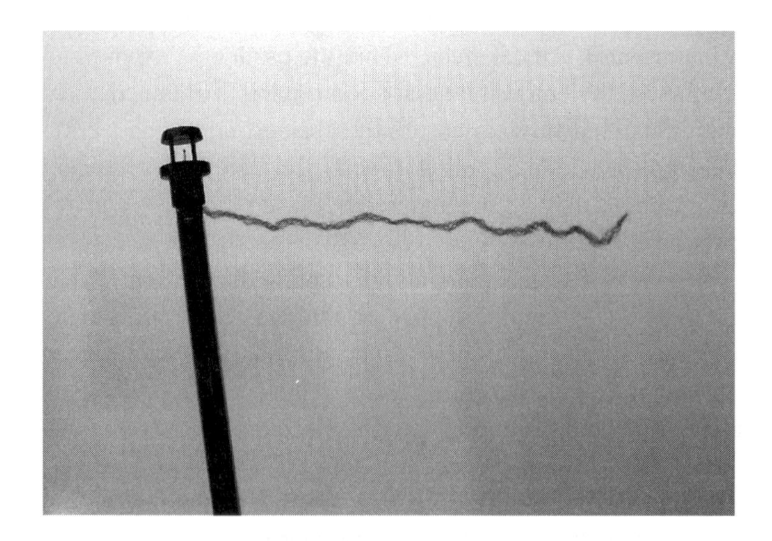

Figure 11.2 Nylon thread streamer used with an anemometer

Streamers are useful to indicate the direction of airflow, but do not give an exact representation; because of their weight steamers do not flow with the air stream. This is a problem that increases as the air velocity decreases. A horizontal flow of air with a velocity of about 0.5 m/s (100 ft/min) is required to get a typical streamer to stream at 45° to the horizontal and a velocity of about 1m/s (200 ft/min) for it to stream almost horizontal.

11.2.1.2 Smoke or particle streams

There are a number of methods suitable for generating smoke or particle streams that are used to show the flow of air in cleanrooms. For example, the apparatus used to produce smoke for testing filter integrity can be used. However, the use of oil smoke may not be acceptable in some cleanrooms, as oil left on surfaces can be a contamination hazard.

Water vapour is a contamination-free alternative and can be produced by different techniques such as from solid CO_2 (dry ice) or by nebulizing water. Figure 11.3 is a photograph of a nebulizing apparatus producing water vapour.

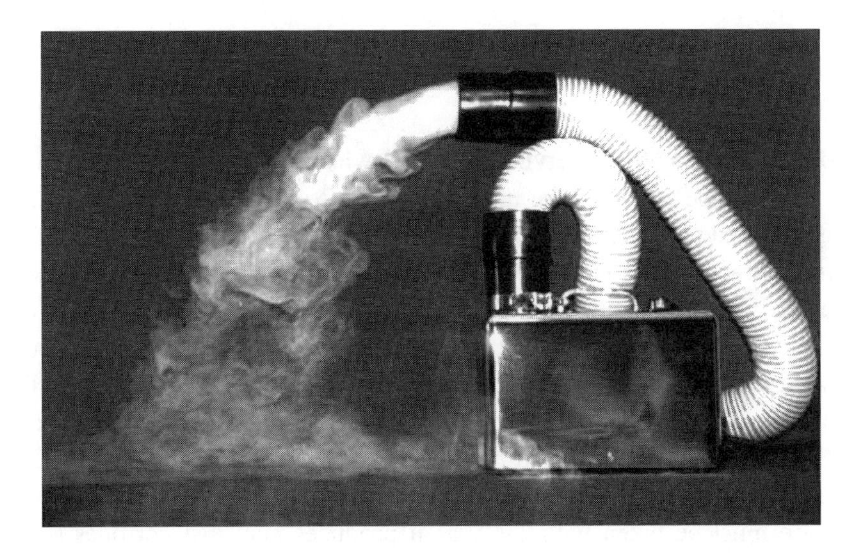

Figure 11.3 Fogger producing water vapour

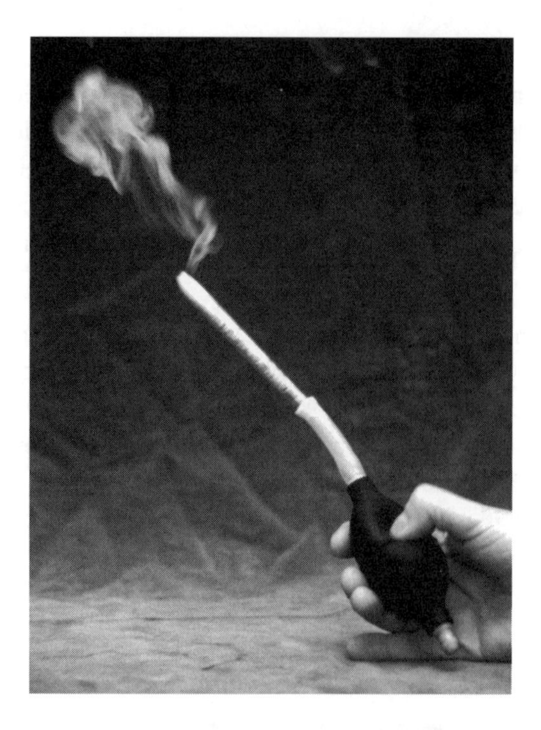

Figure 11.4 Smoke from a puffer

Another technique for observing airflow is what is often known as a 'puffer and smoke tube'. The smoke tubes are about 2 cm in diameter and 10 cm long and made of glass. Within the tube is pumice stone is loaded with Titanium tetrachloride ($TiCl_4$). When required for use, both ends of the glass tube are broken off and one placed into an air puffer. By pressing the puffer, white smoke is expelled through the other end of the tube (Figure 11.4). It is possible to puff smoke in the area to be checked and observe the smoke movement. Titanium tetrachloride can also be purchased in bulk in bottles; bud swabs dipped into it will fume with smoke and can be used to observe air movements.

Care must be taken with $TiCl_4$ as it produces acid that corrodes some surfaces and is likely to be harmful to sensitive machinery. It should not be used when products are exposed in the cleanroom. It is also necessary to ensure that the acid fumes do not harm the operator's lungs.

Using one of the generating methods described above, the airflow in the room can be visualised and areas found where the air movement is poor. Single 'puffs', 'streams' or 'multiple streams' can do this. Sufficient information may be obtained by witnessing the air movement, but a permanent record can be preserved by the use of a video camera.

It will be found in turbulently ventilated rooms that test streams will be quickly dispersed into the cleanroom. If this is so, it demonstrates that the room is working well. Areas where the smoke does not disperse quickly are areas where contamination can build up. These should not occur where the product is exposed to contamination. If necessary, the flow of air can be improved by adjusting the air supply diffuser blades, removing an obstruction, moving a machine, or by some similar solution.

In most cleanrooms the critical area where the product is exposed to contamination will be within a unidirectional flow; this is where the room may be of a unidirectional flow type, or a unidirectional cabinet or workstation is used. In unidirectional flow, air moves in lines and the test stream is much easier to see than in turbulent flow. In unidirectional flow the air coming from the filters should, ideally, flow unimpeded to the critical area. However, problems of the type discussed in section 11.2 may occur. Whether one or more of these problems are likely to cause an unacceptable increase in contamination can be assessed by visualisation techniques.

A useful method of visualisation uses a pipe of about 2.5 cm (1 inch) diameter with 2 to 3 mm diameter holes bored in line, about every 10 cm (4 inches). The pipe is set up on stands and supplied with a smoke stream from a generator. The continuous smoke streams issuing out of the pipe holes gives good visualisation of the unidirectional airflow.

Still pictures can be taken of the airflow, but because of the diffusion of the smoke they are generally not very clear. A video taken of the smoke movement gives the best representation of the airflow. The video pictures can be improved if the room lighting is switched off and the smoke highlighted with columns of light.

11.2.1.3 Air velocity and direction

A permanent record of the airflow within the cleanroom can be obtained by measurement of the velocity and direction over a section of the room. Setting up a grid in the room helps with this. Stands the height of the room should be used and strong thread, such as 4 pound nylon used by fishermen, strung across the stands.

The thread is marked at given intervals, e.g. 10 or 20 cm (4 inches or 8 inches), so that points are available for measuring air velocity and direction. Measurement can be done using a multidirectional anemometer that will give the air velocity either in the X and Y-axis, or in the X, Y and Z-axis. These anemometers can be expensive and a simple anemometer with a streamer attached to give the air direction will give reasonable results, especially if the airflow is unidirectional and reasonably represented in two dimensions.

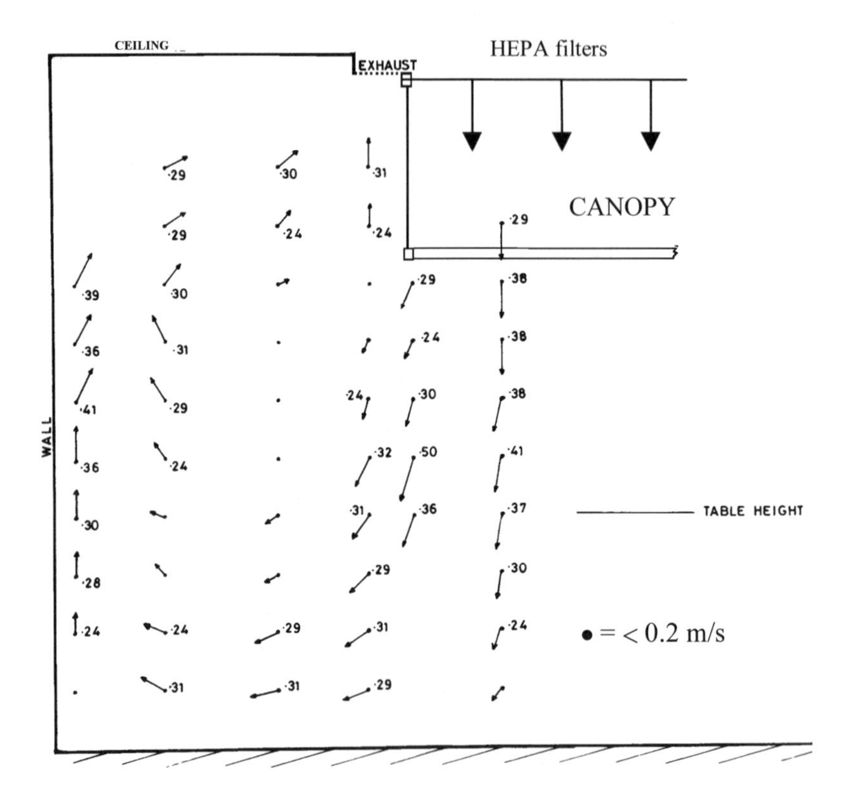

Figure 11.5 The direction and velocity of air coming from the supply filters to the exhaust of a partial-wall unidirectional workstation

Figure 11.5 shows a two dimensional representation of the velocity and direction of unidirectional airflow coming out from a unidirectional workstation. This system had a filter supply area 3m × 3m (10 ft x 10 ft) and walls that stopped 2m (6ft) from the floor, rather than coming down to near the floor. The air exhaust was in the ceiling around the outside of the canopy. Only half of the system is shown. The length of the arrows shown in the figure denotes the magnitude of the air velocity.

This drawing showed that air reaches the table, and the air flow path to the exhaust prevents contamination from outside the workstation area being entrained into the clean area, and hence contaminating any work being carried out around the table.

11.3 Recovery Test Method

The procedures described above are qualitative methods used to show that sufficient clean air gets to the critical areas. A quantitative approach can also be used.

If test particles are introduced into an area being studied, the rate at which they are removed is dependent on the effectiveness of the airflow; the better the air movement and the more air that gets into the test area, the faster the reduction in the particle count.

A burst of test particles should be introduced into the area to be tested, and after the particles have mixed with their surroundings, the airborne particle count should be measured, and at regular intervals. A useful endpoint is one-hundredth of the original concentration, and the time taken to reach there can be used as an index of efficiency. However, this method is dependent on no particles being generated within, or introduced into, the test area; this must be demonstrated before starting the test

Acknowledgement

Figure 11.3 is reproduced by permission of Clean Air Solutions.

12

Filter Installation Leak Testing

As part of the cleanroom testing programme it is necessary to determine that the *quality* of air supplied to a cleanroom is suitable for the task being carried out in the room. High efficiency filters should efficiently remove the particles in the supply air. The filter efficiency will have been defined in the cleanroom design specification and will not be discussed in this chapter (see Chapter 8 for information).

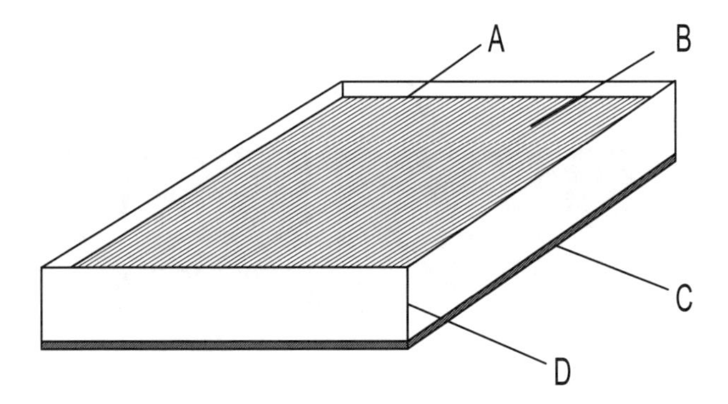

A - filter paper-to-case cement area

C - gasket

D - frame joints.

B - filter paper (often at the paper fold)

Figure 12.1 Leakage areas in a high efficiency filter

High efficiency filters to be installed in the cleanroom will have been tested in the manufacturer's factory and packed so they should arrive at the construction site undamaged. This is not always so. Damage may also occur when the filters are unpacked and fitted into the filter housings. The typical fault areas of an installed filter are shown in Figure 12.1, and these will allow contaminated air to leak through the filter and into the cleanroom.

There can be additional leakage problems associated with the housing into which a filter is fitted; this depends on how the filter is fitted. If the filter is inserted from the top down, i.e. from above the ceiling (Figure 12.2), then the gasket may leak. However, if the filter is inserted from the bottom up i.e. from the cleanroom, the gasket may leak but additional leaks can come from the filter casing (Figure 12.3); the problem of distinguishing between these leaks is discussed later.

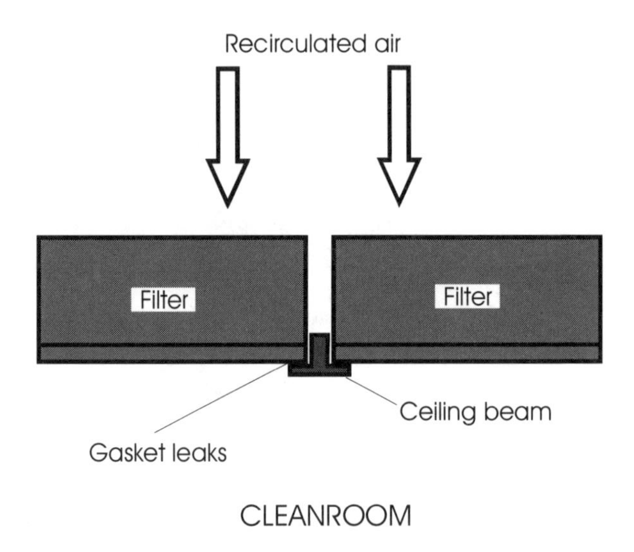

Figure 12.2 Gasket leaks from filters inserted down from ceiling

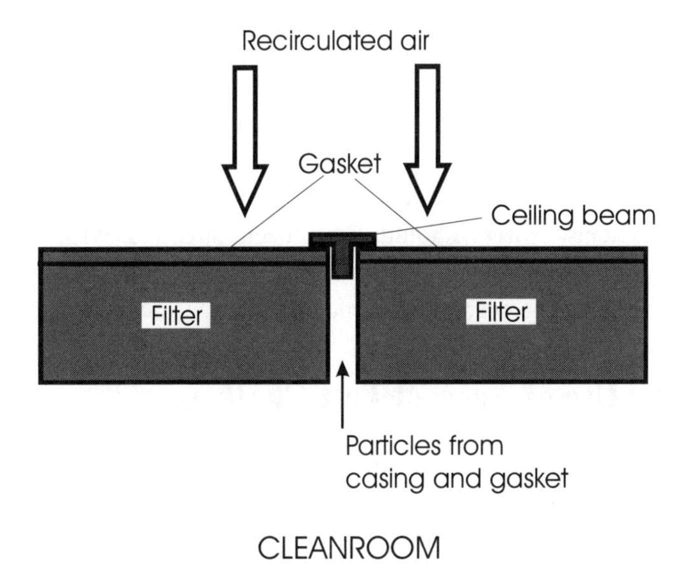

Figure 12.3 Gasket and casing leaks from filter inserted up from cleanroom

A filter housing of the type shown in Figure 12.4 uses gel seals; these will prevent gasket leaks. However, they are more expensive. This type of housing is discussed in Section 8.6 , and is also shown in Figure 8.7.

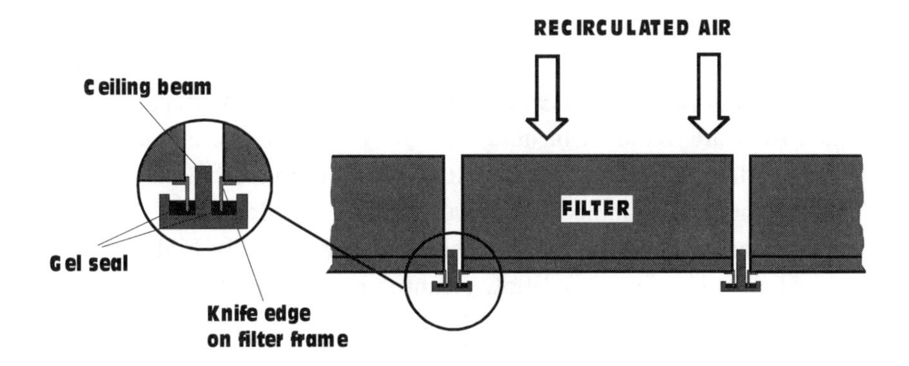

Figure 12.4 Filter-housing gel seal method

Testing a high efficiency filter and its filter housing for leaks is normally done with an artificial test aerosol. This is generated by a dust or smoke generator and injected into the ductwork system so that there is a suitable concentration behind the high efficiency filter. Any problems are found by scanning the filter system for test particles that leak through.

High efficiency filters should have been supplied with the correct particle removal efficiency. A secondary function of the installation leak test is to check that the correct efficiency of filter has been supplied.

12.1 The Use of Aerosol Test Challenges

Before discussing the choice of artificial test aerosols that are available to test filters, it is appropriate to consider two questions. Firstly, is it always necessary to carry out filter leakage tests in cleanrooms, and secondly, is an artificial test challenge necessary?

It is fairly common in poorer quality cleanrooms [occasionally in ISO Class 7 (Class 10 000) and frequently in ISO Class 8 (Class 100 000)] not to carry out filter integrity tests. ISO Class 8 (Class 100 000) rooms may not use high efficiency filters in a terminal position in the supply duct, but bag-type filters positioned after the air conditioning plant; it will not then be possible to carry out a leak test of the type described in this chapter. It is also argued that if the air classification standard is achieved within the cleanroom then a small leakage of unfiltered air through the filter system has had little influence and is acceptable. This viewpoint is quite acceptable in turbulently ventilated rooms where the supply air is well mixed with the room air, and localised concentrations of contamination arising from a damaged filter are avoided. In unidirectional flow systems, especially in a cabinet or isolator where the distance from the filter to the critical area may be small, a hole in a faulty filter could give a unidirectional stream of contamination; this may give a localised and unacceptably high counts at the critical area. Unidirectional flow cleanrooms, and clean air devices that use unidirectional airflow, are therefore always tested for filter faults.

In some cleanrooms, an artificial test challenge is not used to test the filters but the normal particle load in the supply air is used instead. It is argued that if the filter is tested for leaks with a particle counter (not a photometer) and no significant particle concentrations are detected, then there is no need to test the filter with abnormally high concentrations of particles. A reason given against this argument is that filter tests are normally carried out when the room is empty. The air recirculated from the empty room will therefore have fewer particles than the occupied room. However, it is possible to overcome this problem by using outside fresh air, as this has a high particle concentration. If the fresh air is filtered with high efficiency filters then these should be removed. The percentage of recirculated air should also be cut back as much as possible, so that the dilution of fresh air particles is minimised. This air may then give a sufficiently high concentration of particle challenge to find any filter leakage that will contribute to the particle count in the room.

The choice as to whether or not to use an artificial test challenge may not be an open one, but determined by the requirement to conform to a cleanroom standard; this means that a test challenge is normally required.

12.2 Artificial Smoke and Particle Test Challenges

The following artificial aerosols are available for testing filter installations in cleanrooms.

12.2.1 Cold-generated oils

Di-octyl phthalate (DOP) is an oily liquid previously used to test filters. Because of potentially toxic effects, it is no longer used in many countries and similar oils, such as di-octylsebacate (DOS), Shell Ondina mineral oil, poly alpha olefin (PAO) or di-ethyl hexylsebacate (DEHS) are used.

To create a cold-generated test aerosol, air is passed at high pressure through a nozzle designed for this purpose known as a Laskin nozzle. The air exits from the nozzle at high velocity and as it does so it shears the oil drawn from the reservoir. Fine particles of a mass median diameter of about 0.5 μm are ejected at a small positive pressure. These test particles should be introduced into the air supply at a position sufficiently removed from the filters to give good mixing and hence an even concentration across the back of the filter.

The output of one Laskin nozzle is relatively small (about 0.4g/min) and is only sufficient to test challenge a small volume ventilation system. The air volume that can be tested will depend on the concentration of the test challenge used, but a system supplying about 0.5 m^3/s (1000 ft^3/min) of air can be tested when the filter penetration is measured by a photometer. Multiple nozzle systems are therefore necessary for a larger volume system if a photometer is used.

Another possibility is to use a single particle counter in place of a photometer. According to the IEST RP CC006, a concentration of 10 μg/l of test aerosol will give a count of about 3×10^{10} $/m^3$ ($10^9/ft^3$) of particles produced by a Laskin nozzle, and so a particle counter should be able to deal with most cleanrooms. Another alternative is to use of a photometer with a generator that produces larger quantities of test challenge by a hot generated method.

12.2.2 Hot generated smokes

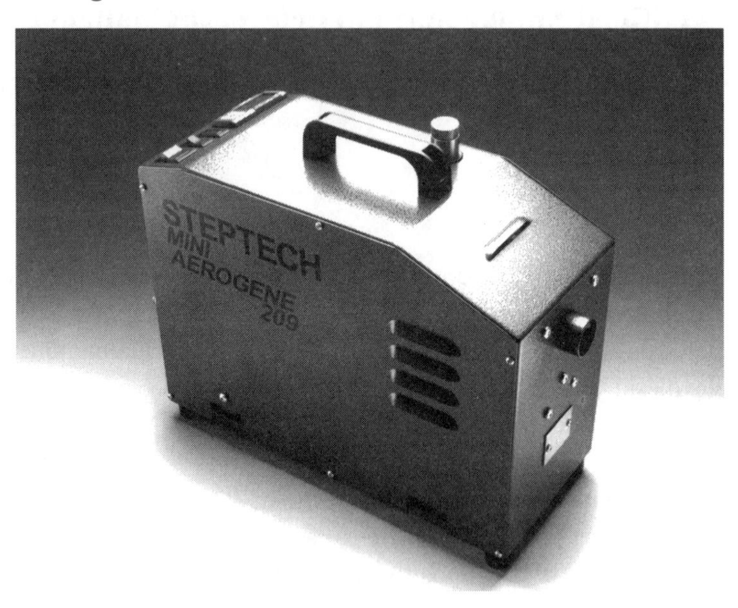

Figure 12.5 Hot oil smoke generator

Because of the difficulty of generating sufficient challenge from Laskin nozzles, hot-generated test smokes are often used. These also have the advantage of requiring no air pumps; Laskin nozzles in a multi-nozzle format require an impractical amount of air for what must be a portable system. These thermal generators use an inert gas, such as CO_2, to inject suitable oil into a heated evaporation chamber. The vaporised oil is then condensed as a fine aerosol of a mass median diameter of about 0.3 μm at the exit nozzle.

Generators of the type shown in Figure 12.5 will produce around 10 to 50 g/min of aerosol, this being sufficient to test (in association with a photometer) an air ventilation system of up to about 40 m^3/s (85 000 ft^3/min).

12.2.3 Polystyrene latex spheres

In some cleanroom situations, such as semiconductor manufacturing, inert test particles are specified. This is done to ensure that there is no possibility of 'outgassing' of chemical products harmful to the process from any test aerosol left on the filter. Outside air has been used for this purpose, but the test particle of choice, at the moment, is Polystyrene Latex Spheres (PLSs). These are available in a wide range of monodispersed solutions from 0.1 to 1 μm in size, so that an appropriate size can be chosen. These solutions are aerosolised and measured by a particle counter.

12.3 Apparatus for Measuring Smoke Penetration

12.3.1 Photometer

A typical photometer will draw 28 l/min (1 ft^3/min) of airborne particles into it. These pass through a sample tube and across an area where light is concentrated. Particles refract the light and this light passes through a collecting lens and onto a photomultiplier tube where the light is converted into an electrical signal.

Photometers usually measure a particle concentration of between 0.0001 μg/l and 100 μg/l. Such readings are dependent not only on the number of particles but their size, i.e. their *mass*. A typical photometer is shown in Figure 12.6.

A photometer has an advantage over the single particle counter in that the concentration challenge can be measured, and this reading, by a flick of the switch, can then become the 100% reading. The instrument is then switched to an appropriate scale and when the leak penetration through the filter, e.g. 0.01% is exceeded this can be shown on the scale, or by an audible alarm.

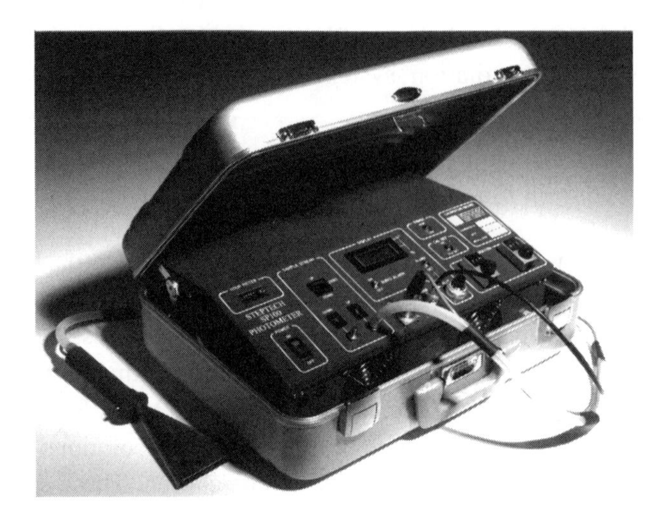

Figure 12.6 A typical photometer

12.3.2 Single particle counters

Particle counters of the type normally used to count and size particles in the air of cleanrooms can be used to carry out filter leak testing. However, the particle counter must be able to run in a continuous measuring mode. Particle counters are normally used to sample a volume of air and this is collected in a set time; some counters do not therefore sample continuously. If a particle counter is used to measure leaks in filters, the upstream particle challenge count is likely to be higher than the range of the instrument and can cause contamination problems in the instrument. A device will have to be purchased to dilute the upstream sample.

12.4 Methods of Testing Filters and Filter Housings

12.4.1 Scanning methods

Before starting to test the integrity of filters, it will be necessary to consider smoke alarms. Smoke leaking round the generator, especially if it is brought into the cleanroom to test clean air devices can set off smoke alarms. The possibilities and consequences of smoke alarms going off should be considered. It is best to turn them off during the test period rather than suffer the embarrassment of the arrival of the fire brigade, or a dousing from water sprinklers.

The normal scanning method is to use a probe together with a photometer, or single particle counter, to scan over the whole filter face. The perimeter of the filter is then scanned for leaks between the filter media and its filter case, and the filter case and its housing. The probe is normally held about 2.5 cm (1 inch) from the filter and the filter scanned with overlapping strokes (Figure 12.7).

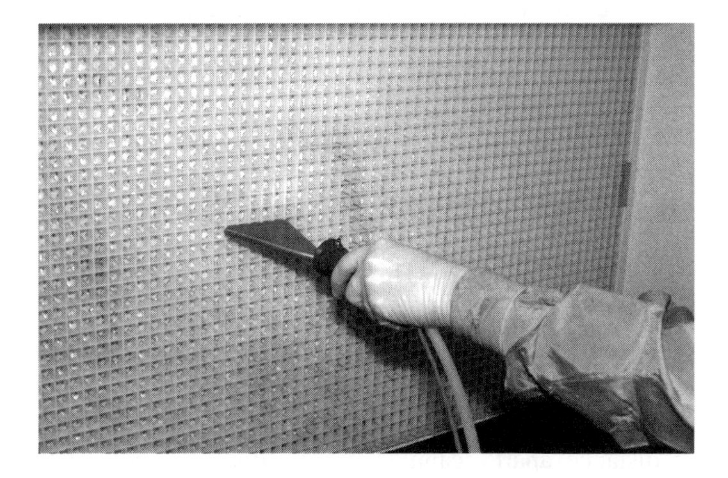

Figure 12.7 Scanning a filter

The speed of scan is important. If the probe passes slowly over a hole it will pick up more particles and find more faults. A quick run over the filter will not be sufficient to pick up some faults, and this should be guarded against. A scan speed of not more than 5cm/s is reasonable but the IEST RP CC006 gives a method by which a more scientific approach can be used to ascertain the scan speed.

If a photometer is used, the concentration of the challenge smoke is measured behind the filter and adjusted to a suitable concentration. This concentration will depend on the acceptable leakage. If it is 0.01% of the challenge then a concentration of about 10 μg/l is reasonable. The photometer is then adjusted so that the upstream concentration becomes the 100% reading and the percentage penetration is then read directly from the photometer scale. If a concentration of test challenge exceeds 0.01% of the contamination generated behind the filter, it is then considered as a leak.

The most common leaks are around the periphery of the filter. They may come from the casing-to-housing seal, or when the filter is inserted from the cleanroom side, the casing joints as well (see Figures 12.2 and 12.3). In the former case, the filter will probably have to be removed and re-seated correctly. In the case of a room-inserted filter, it is difficult to distinguish between a casing and a casing-to-housing leak. It may be necessary to check for casing leaks on a rig, re-fit, and check for housing leaks.

12.4.2 Testing filters in unidirectional flow rooms

The problem with checking the filter bank in the ceiling of a unidirectional flow room is that the air filter area is so large that testing will take a considerable amount of time. This may be several days for a large semiconductor fabrication cleanroom. It may be useful to use methods that reduce the time. It is possible to use several particle sampler sensors of the type shown in Figure 13.6 in Chapter 13. By placing them on a motorised trolley with their inlet nozzles at a suitable height from the filter bank, and the correct distance apart, scanning can be done by moving the trolley about the room. The scanning time can therefore be substantially reduced.

It is also possible to scan each filter, and its casing, on a rig in the cleanroom and then carefully take the scanned filter, and place it into its housing in the ceiling. It is then only necessary to check the periphery of the filters for filter-to-housing leaks when the whole filter ceiling is in place and the ventilation system switched on.

12.4.3 Filter testing in conventionally ventilated room

A conventionally ventilated room will generally be ISO Class 4 (Class 1000), or poorer. The products manufactured within the room are therefore unlikely to be susceptible to oil out-gassing from the air filter, and oil smoke can be used as a test challenge. Photometers are therefore most commonly used. To obtain good mixing, the test smoke should be injected well up the ductwork system away from the filter. Introducing it into the ventilation plant at a point before the fan will give good mixing. If there is any doubt as to the thoroughness of the mixing, its uniformity behind the filter should be checked. If an air diffuser is fitted after the filter, this should be removed to give access to the filter surface. Scanning of the filter is then carried out.

12.4.4 Repair of leaks

If a leak is found to be coming from the filter media, it is often at the fold of the paper. This can be repaired on site with silicon mastic and it is generally accepted that a small area of the filter area can be repaired. However, if no repairs are acceptable and imperfect filters must be replaced, then this should be agreed with the contractor at the quotation stage, as a quotation that includes the removal and replacement of filters is likely to be more expensive.

Acknowledgement

Figures 12.5 and 12.6 are reproduced by permission of Steptech Instrument Services.

13

Airborne Particle Counts

The most important test used to ensure a cleanroom is working correctly is a count of the airborne particles. Before proceeding with this count, the tests described in Chapters 9 to 12 should have been carried out on the following; the air supply volume, the pressure differences, the air movement within and between cleanrooms, and the filter integrity. These should all have been demonstrated to be satisfactory. It is then necessary, as a final test, to show that the airborne particle concentration does not exceed the particle class limit in the agreed occupancy state, or states.

13.1 Airborne Particle Counters

An instrument known as a 'particle counter' is used to count and size particles in the air of a cleanroom. This is often called a 'single particle counter' to distinguish it from a photometer used to test filter installation leakage. A particle counter both counts and sizes particles in the air, whereas a photometer simply measures the mass of particles. For the sake of simplicity, the former instrument is called in this chapter a 'particle counter'.

A particle counter is an essential tool for testing and running cleanrooms. Good second hand models are often available at a modest price, so that no cleanroom should be without one. Figure 13.1 shows a typical particle counter. Particle counters of this type, size particles in the range of 0.3–10 µm. Airborne particle counters will normally sample 28 l/min (1 ft^3/min) of air and are available in models that size particles down to either 0.3 µm or 0.5 µm. Some high-sensitivity models can count down to about 0.1µm, but often with a smaller air sampling volume.

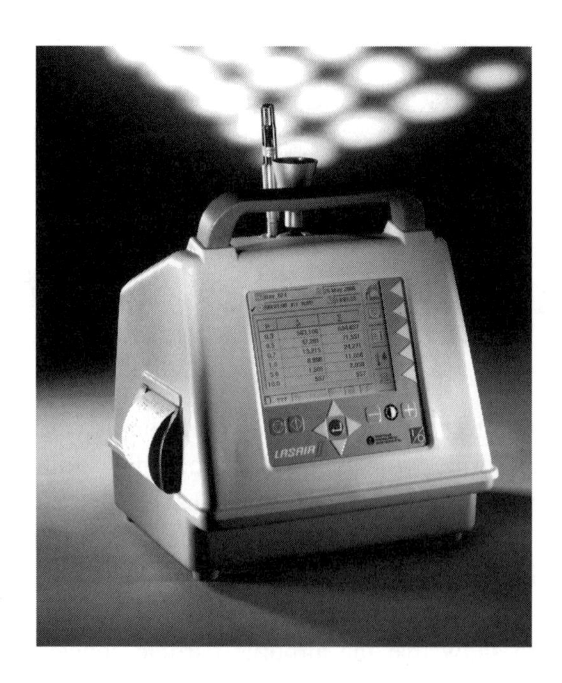

Figure 13.1 Airborne particle counter

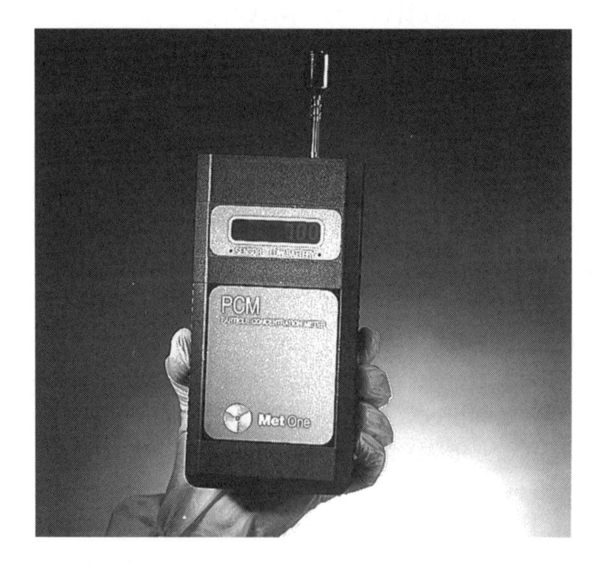

Figure 13.2 Hand-held particle counter

It is possible to purchase hand-held models of the type shown in Figure 13.2. Because of the amount of electrical power required, hand-held models may only sample 2.8 l/min (0.1ft^3/min) of air and size down to 0.5 μm.

Figure 13.3 shows how a particle counter works. It uses a photodiode to sense light scattered by single particles passing through a beam of light in a sensing zone. The light source is typically a laser diode or, for greater sensitivity, a HeNe laser. The scattered light is concentrated by a lens system and converted by the photodiode into electrical pulses, their amplitude being in proportion to the particle size. Thus, the size of particle can be measured.

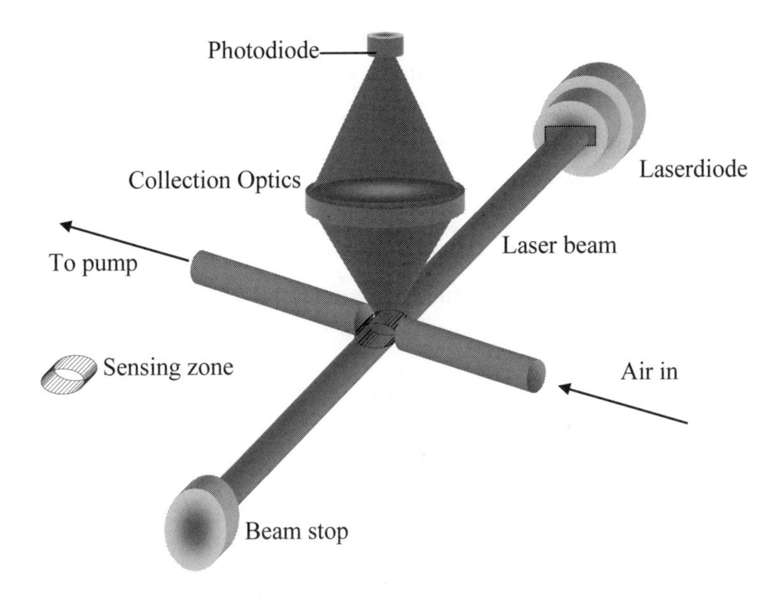

Figure 13.3 Detection method used in a particle counter

The instrument can also count the number of pulses produced by the photodiode, and hence the number of particles is ascertained. Particles are normally counted on a 'equal to and greater' size basis, and all particles equal and greater to a given size are counted. This method of measurement is the same as specified in the cleanroom standards.

13.2 Continuous Monitoring Apparatus for Airborne Particles

In high quality cleanrooms, where the product is very susceptible to airborne particle contamination, continuous monitoring of the air is used to check for deviations from the required airborne particle cleanliness. However, in lesser quality cleanrooms it is not necessary to sample continuously; a technician moving a particle counter about the cleanroom can carry out the testing. However, the technician's time is expensive, and their presence adds to the airborne contamination in the room. It is sometimes better to continuously monitor the particle count.

There are two main methods of continuous sampling. These are often called 'sequential' and 'simultaneous'. In a *sequential monitoring* system, as shown in Figure 13.4, the room is fitted with sampling tubes and a sample of air is taken from each sampling point in turn. This air is transported through sampling tubes, via a manifold, to a particle counter, where the particles are counted. To add to the efficiency of the operation, the results are usually analysed.

The *simultaneous monitoring* system, of the type shown in Figure 13.5, uses many small sensors to continuously size and count particles in the air at various points of the room.

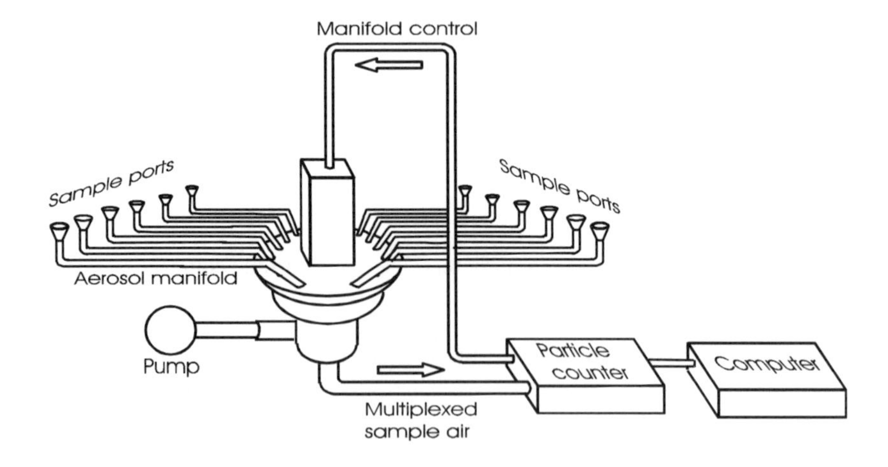

Figure 13.4 Sequential monitoring system

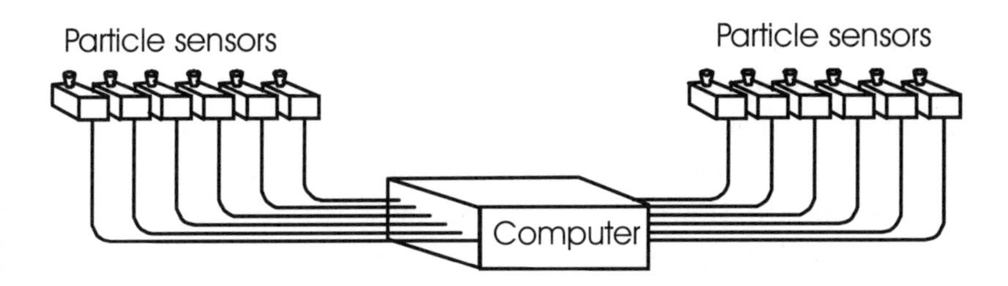

Figure 13.5 Simultaneous monitoring system

Figure 13.6 shows a typical sensor, its size being compared to a pencil. Information on the number and size of airborne particles measured by sensors is transmitted by electrical signals through a cable to a computer where they are analysed.

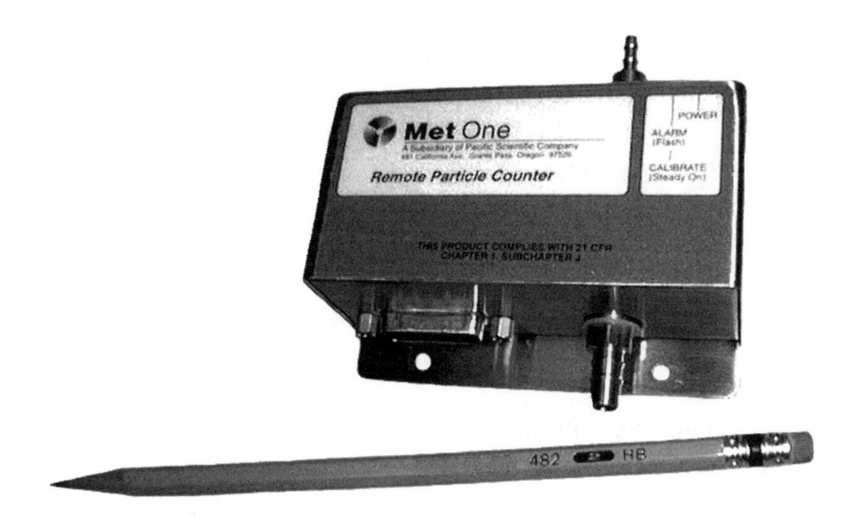

Figure 13.6 Sensor used in simultaneous sampling

Both monitoring systems use software packages to analyse the results. These can establish the overall average count in the room of various particle sizes, or calculate average counts at each position in the room.

They can also register any results that are greater than an 'alert' or 'action' value set into the computer. Other information can also be made available.

It would appear that the simultaneous monitoring system is the best system, as air is continuously sampled at the chosen sampling places and no high counts missed. However, it is also the most expensive system. The sequential method deposits particles on the inner surfaces of the tubing that runs to the particle sampler, as well as within the manifold. However, these losses on the inner tube surfaces can be minimised if care is taken in the design of the system. If small particles ($\leq$ 5 μm) are measured, the losses caused by deposition are small and usually acceptable; it is, after all, increases in particle counts that are sought rather than absolute values.

13.3 Particle Counting in Different Occupancy States

One of the final tasks that must be carried out, prior to hand-over of the cleanroom to the user, is the measurement of the airborne particle concentration. This is done to ensure that the count is within the standards set down at the design stage.

The airborne contamination in a cleanroom can be measured in three occupancy states. These are defined in ISO 14664-1 as:

- *As built*: complete and ready for operation, with all services connected and functional, but without equipment or operating personnel in the facility;
- *At rest:* complete, with all services functioning and with equipment installed and operable or operating, as specified, but without operating personnel in the facility;
- *Operational:* in normal operation, with all services functioning and with equipment and personnel, if applicable, present and performing their normal work functions in the facility.

There can often be a considerable time delay between the cleanroom being completed by the building contractor and products being manufactured in the room. However, the contractor will wish to be paid for building the cleanroom and it is common practice to check that the room in its 'as-built' condition is satisfactory, and if it is, to pay all or most of the fee. The problem with checking the 'as-built' condition is that as there is no equipment working, nor personnel in the room, there is no generation of airborne particles. Thus, the airborne particle concentration can be very close to that of the filtered air supply. In practice, one or more people are required to test the room and they will increase the particle count. However, the particle count will be much lower than when the room is 'operational'.

It will be to the advantage of the cleanroom contractor to have the class limits confirmed in the 'as built' occupancy state. The 'as built' state should have the lowest count of all the occupancy states, and this can be tested as soon as the room is ready. If the occupancy state has not been specified in the building contract there may be problems. The user may wish the cleanroom to perform satisfactorily in the occupied state, whereas the contractor may consider the room gives the correct class, albeit in the 'at rest' state. It should therefore be made clear in the building contract what occupancy state should apply.

If a cleanroom has been designed properly and the cleanroom tested when empty, i.e. in the 'as-built' state then there is a 'rule of thumb' assumption that can be applied. This is that the 'as built' room will be about one class of cleanliness cleaner than when 'operational'. This is not always correct, but it should be possible, by the use of some additional tests in the 'as-built' state, to predict how likely it is to conform to the class limit in either the 'at-rest' or 'operational' state. The important confirmatory tests are the quality and quantity of air supplied. Because of the directed airflow in a unidirectional system, the correct standards are likely to be achieved if the filters have no particles by-passing them, and the air velocities are correct. In a turbulently ventilated room, the achievement of the correct standard in its 'operational' state is less certain, as it is dependant on the air supply volume being sufficient to dilute the contamination dispersed from machines and people. However, this should not be a problem if an experienced designer is used. It is more normal to find that the designer over-designs and the cleanroom ends up cleaner than expected.

After the contractor has handed over the cleanroom, the equipment will be installed and commissioned and, finally, production will start. The particle contamination can then be measured at the 'operational' state. The 'operational' condition is the most relevant condition to be measured, as it reflects the actual contamination when the manufacturing area is working; this condition is also likely to give the highest particle count.

13.4 Measurement of Particle Concentrations (ISO 14644-1)

The standard of a cleanroom is defined by the concentration of airborne particles, at a given size or sizes, that is not to be exceeded in a given occupancy state. These class limits are calculated by use of Equation 3.1 in Section 3.4 of this book. Some typical class limits for various particle sizes are given in Table 3.2, and also in Figure 3.2 in Chapter 3.

To classify a cleanroom, it is necessary to take sufficient samples of air to have confidence that the airborne particle concentration of the room is within the limits set by the standards. The number of sampling locations must reflect the size of the room and its cleanliness. The larger and cleaner the room, the more sampling locations that must be used. The air sample must also be of a sufficiently large volume to give confidence in the results. The methods for (a) selection of the number of sampling locations and (b) determining the minimum air volume are laid down in ISO 14644-1, and explained below. The acceptance criteria that must be met for a cleanroom to achieve a given classification are given in the ISO 14644-1 and described below. Similar methods are used within the Federal Standard 209 E, and where these deviate from the ISO method, it is pointed out. However, anyone wishing to test a cleanroom must purchase the relevant standards (see Section 4.2.1.3 for information.)

13.4.1 Sample locations and number

ISO standard 14644-1 gives a formula by which the minimum number of locations can be calculated. This is as follows:

$$N_L = \sqrt{A} \qquad (13.1)$$

where,
N_L is the minimum number of sampling locations (rounded up to a whole number)
and A is the area of the cleanroom, or clean air controlled space, in m^2.

The ISO standard requires that the samples are evenly distributed around the cleanroom and placed at a height where the work is carried out. The method outlined in Federal Standard 209 E for calculating the number of sampling locations are substantially different from the ISO standard. These calculations depend on whether the cleanroom is unidirectional or non-unidirectional. To obtain fuller information, Federal Standard 209 E should be consulted. If the method given in Federal Standard 209 E is used it will give a larger number of sample locations than that suggested in the ISO 14644-1 standard. Federal Standard 209 E is, in my opinion, over-generous and the ISO requirements are more appropriate.

13.4.2 Airborne sampling volume

It is necessary to determine the minimum volume of air to be sampled at each location. Because there are fewer particles in cleaner rooms, a larger air sample will be required to be confident that the results are within particle class limits given in the standards. Both the ISO 14644-1 and Federal Standard 209 E standards require that the air volume should be large enough to count 20 particles of the largest particle size specified, if the concentration was at the class limit being considered.

The following formula is used to calculate the minimum volume:

$$V = \frac{20}{C} \times 1000$$

where,
V is the minimum single sample volume per location, expressed in litres.
C is the class limit (number of particles/m^3) for the largest considered particle size specified for the relevant class.
20 is the defined number of particles that could be counted if the particle concentration were at the class limit.

One or more samples can be taken at each location. The volume sampled at each location should be at least two litres, and the minimum sample time should be at least one minute.

13.4.3 Acceptance criteria

The ISO standard 14644-1 considers that a cleanroom has met the required classification if:

1. the average particle concentration at each of the particle measuring locations falls below the class limit;
2. when the total number of locations sampled is less than 10, the calculated 95% Upper Confidence Limit (UCL) of the particle concentrations is below the class limit.

The Federal Standard 209 E standard sets almost identical requirements.

13.5 Worked Example of ISO 14644-1 Test Method

To show the application of the ISO 14644-1 method, the following is taken as an example:

A cleanroom is 4m × 5m in floor size. It should comply with ISO Class 3 in the 'as built' condition at a particle size of ≥ 0.1 μm.

The calculations are as follows.

13.5.1 Number of locations

The area of the cleanroom floor is 4m × 5m. Therefore, the number of sampling locations = $\sqrt{4 \times 5} = 4.47$

The minimum number of locations, rounded up to the nearest whole number, is therefore 5. Had the room been required to comply with FS 209 E a different calculation would have been needed. That calculation would depend on whether the room was unidirectional or nonunidirectional.

13.5.2 Minimum air sampling volume

$$\text{The minimum volume (particle size} \geq 0.1\ \mu\text{m)} = \frac{20}{\text{class limit for the given particle size}} \times 1000$$

The class limit for a particle size of $\geq$ 0.1 μm in an ISO Class 3 room is $1000/\text{m}^3$.

$$\therefore \text{Minimum volume} = \frac{20}{1000} \times 1000 = 20\ \text{litres}$$

Using a particle counter with a sampling rate of 28.3 l, i.e. 1 ft /min, a 42 second sample will be required for each location. However, ISO 14644-1 requires a minimum sample time of 1 minute.

13.5.3 Sampling results

Five locations must be sampled to fulfil the requirements laid down in the ISO 14644-1 standard. A sample set of results is given in Table 13.1.

Table 13.1 Particle counts at locations in the cleanroom

Sampling Location	Number of particles $\geq$ 0.1 μm /28 litres	Number of particles $\geq$ 0.1 μm /m^3
1	12	580
2	22	612
3	20	706
4	15	530
5	10	553

The results given are one minute samples and only one sample is given at each location, although averages of multiple samples or one long sample can be used. All of the results shown are below the class limit for the ISO Class 3 room, i.e. $1000/\text{m}^3$ for particles $\geq$ 0.1 μm. The first part of the ISO requirement is therefore satisfied. If the class limit is exceeded then the

ISO standard accepts that sampling can be performed at additional evenly distributed sampling locations. These results are definitive.

As less than nine samples were taken in our sample, it is now necessary to show that the 95% UCL does not exceeded the class limit. This is done using the following method. Firstly, the 'means of averages' is calculated by the equation:

$$\text{Mean of the averages (M)} = \frac{\text{Sum of individual averages}}{\text{Number of individual averages}}$$

The mean of averages in this example is taken from the individual results, as only one sample has been taken at each location. The value can be calculated as follows:

Mean of the averages for particles ≥ 0.1 μm (M)

$$= \frac{580 + 612 + 706 + 530 + 553}{5} = 596$$

Using a mean of the averages equal to 596 the standard deviation of the means is now calculated as follows:

Standard deviation (s.d.)

$$= \sqrt{\frac{(580 - 596)^2 + (612 - 596)^2 + (706 - 596)^2 + (530 - 596)^2 + (553 - 596)^2}{5 - 1}}$$

$$= \sqrt{\frac{256 + 256 + 12100 + 4356 + 1849}{4}}$$

$= 69$

where 5 in the denominator is the number of sample locations.

The 95% UCL is now calculated.

Table 13.2 t-factor for 95% UCL

Number of Locations	2	3	4	5	6	7-9
95% UCL factor	6.3	2.9	2.4	2.1	2.0	1.9

The 't-factors' used in the calculation are given in Table 13.2. As the number of locations is 5, the UCL t-factor chosen from Table 13.2 is 2.1.

The 95% UCL is now calculated using the equation:

$$95\%\,\text{UCL} = \text{M} + \left[\text{UCL factor} \times \frac{\text{s.d.}}{\sqrt{\text{n}}}\right]$$

where, n = number of individual location averages

$$\therefore\ 95\%\ \text{UCL for particles} \geq 0.1\ \mu\text{m} = 596 + \left[2.1 \times \frac{69}{\sqrt{5}}\right] = 661$$

From these calculations it may be seen that the calculated value of the 95% UCL is less than the required class limit of 1000. The cleanroom is therefore within the required class limit.

The above set of results meet the second part of the ISO 14644-1 acceptance criterion, as the calculated 95% UCL is below the class limit. However, a large variation of the results, or an unusually low (or high) result may cause the 95% UCL to exceed the class limit. An example is five sampling locations that gave counts of 926, 958, 937, 963 and 214. The 95% UCL of these results can be calculated to be 1108 particles/m^3. This cleanroom does not pass the acceptance criterion because of the one *low* result. If such a single 'outlier' is the cause of failure, and the reason can be found, then the ISO standard gives a method to treat and correct this problem. Such reasons are typically a mistake made during the sampling, or a sample point directly under a jet of clean air coming from an air terminal.

The way to avoid any 95% UCL problems is to always test more than nine points in the room; the time involved in additional sampling is often less than that required for the calculation of the 95% UCL.

Acknowledgements

Figure 13.1 is reproduced by permission of Particle Measuring Systems. Figures 13.4 and 13.5 have been redrawn from drawings supplied by Particle Measuring Systems. Figures 13.2 and 13.6 are reproduced by permission of Pacific Scientific Instruments. Bob Latimer of Pacific Scientific Instruments drew Figure 13.3. Extracts of ISO 14644-1 are reproduced by permission of the British Standards Institution.

14

Microbial Counts

In bioclean rooms, such as those used by pharmaceutical and medical device manufacturers, the microbial population, as well as dust particles, have to be controlled. People are normally the only source of micro-organisms in a cleanroom. Testing for micro-organisms in the 'as built' or the 'at rest' operational conditions will therefore be of little value. However, when a cleanroom is fully operational, micro-organisms are continually dispersed from people in the room. It will therefore be necessary to monitor the cleanroom to demonstrate that a pre-determined concentration is not exceeded.

It is common to sample the air and surfaces of the cleanroom, as well as the personnel working in the cleanroom. Examples of the microbial concentrations that should not be exceeded in a cleanroom are given in the EU GGMP (shown in Table 3.4) the FDA 'Guideline on Sterile Drug Products Produced by Aseptic Processing'; both are discussed in Section 3.5.

14.1 Microbial Sampling of the Air

Several types of apparatus exist for counting micro-organisms in the air of cleanrooms. These samplers are sometimes known as 'volumetric' air samplers because a given volume of air is sampled, thus distinguishing them from settle plate sampling, where micro-organisms are deposited, mainly by gravity, onto an agar plate. For a similar reason, this type of sampling is also known as 'active' sampling. Many types of samplers have been invented for sampling micro-organisms in the air. In cleanrooms, the most popular types are those that:

1. impact micro-organisms onto agar media;
2. remove micro-organisms by membrane filtration.

14.1.1 Impaction onto agar.

Impaction samplers commonly used in cleanrooms employ the following techniques to remove micro-organisms from the air:

- inertial impaction
- centrifugal forces.

Both these methods impact the microbe-carrying particles onto an agar surface. Agar is a jelly-type material with nutrients added to support microbial growth. Micro-organisms landing on a nutrient agar surface will multiply. If left at a suitable temperature, for sufficient time, the micro-organisms will have multiplied sufficiently for a colony of a few millimetres diameter to be seen. Bacteria will normally be incubated for 48 hours at 30° C to 35° C; a further 72 hours at 20° C to 25° C will allow fungi to grow. Colonies are counted, and hence the number of micro-organisms that have been deposited can be ascertained.

14.1.1.1 Inertial impaction samplers

These samplers will typically sample 30 to 180 litres/min (approximately 1 ft^3/min to 6 ft^3/min) of air, although one brand of slit sampler can sample up to 700 litres/min (25 ft^3/min). Airborne microbial concentrations of 1 /m^3 and less are measured in a cleanroom. Therefore samplers that sample larger volumes of air reduce the sampling time; a sampling volume of 100 l/min (approximately 3 ft^3/min), or greater, is best.

Inertial impactors accelerate air that contains microbe-carrying particles through a slit or hole. The principle of inertial impaction through a slit is shown in Figure 14.1. The air that passes through a slit or hole is accelerated to a velocity high enough to ensure that as the air turns through 90° the particles leave the air stream (about 20 m/s to 30 m/s). This is caused by their inertia, and they impact onto the agar surface. When incubated at a suitable temperature for a specified time, microbe-carrying particles on the agar will grow to form a microbial colony, which can then

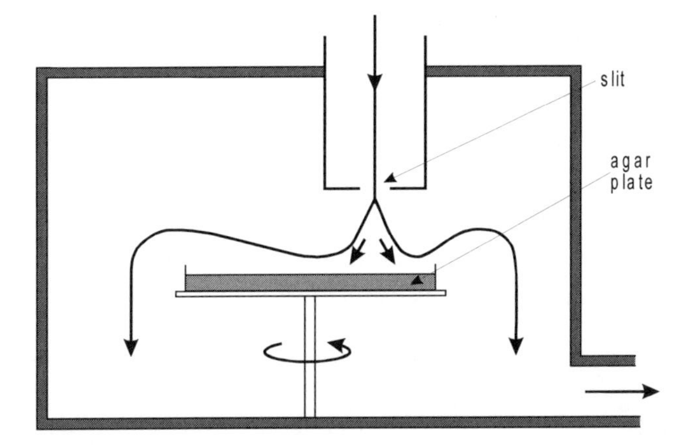

Figure 14.1 Airflow within a slit to agar sampler. Note that both the slit width and distance from the slit-to-agar will be much smaller than shown.

be counted. Thus the number of microbe-carrying particles in a given volume of air can be determined.

A sampler that draws air through multiple holes, i.e. a sieve, and impacts the microbe-carrying particles onto an agar surface is shown in Figure 14.2. The outer sieve with its multiple holes has been removed to show a dish containing agar onto which the microbe containing particles are impacted.

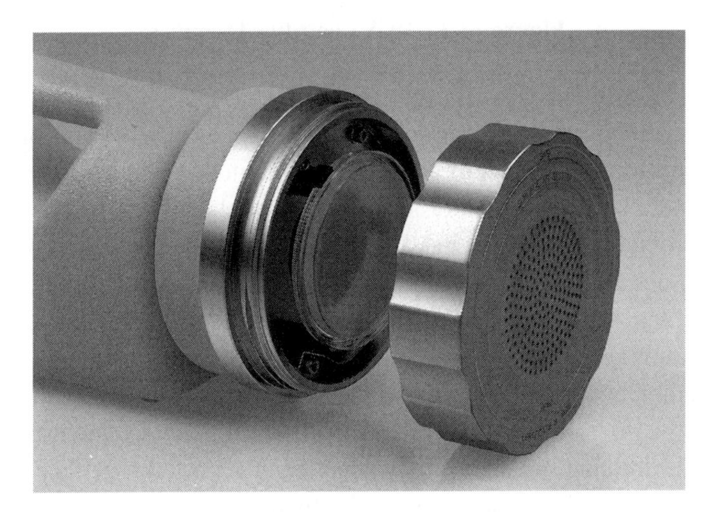

Figure 14.2 SAS air sampler

14.1.1.2 Centrifugal air samplers

An example of a centrifugal sampler is shown in Figure 14.3. In this type of sampler, the air is drawn into the sampler by a rotating vane. This vane then throws, by centrifugal force, the microbe-carrying particles out of the air and onto an agar surface. The impaction surface is in the form of a plastic strip with rectangular recesses into which agar is dispensed. After sampling, the agar strip is removed from the sampler and incubated so that the microbe-containing particles can be ascertained.

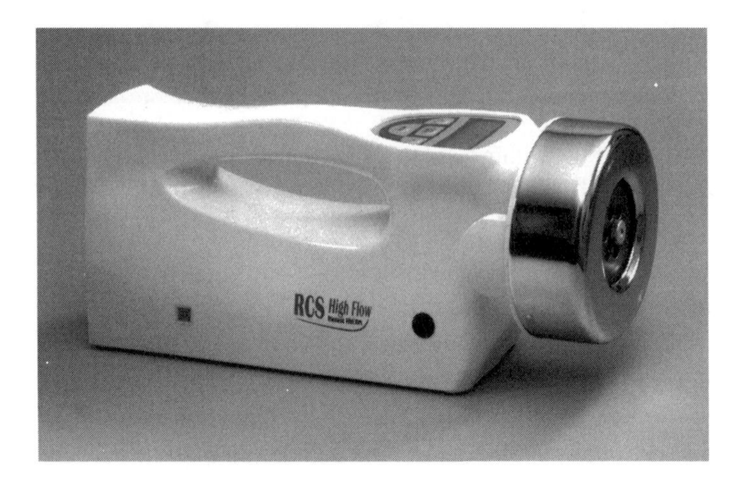

Figure 14.3 RCS Centrifugal sampler

14.1.1.3 Membrane filtration

Another method used to sample micro-organisms in cleanroom air is membrane filtration. A membrane filter is mounted in a holder, a vacuum is applied and a known amount of air drawn through it. The microbe-carrying particles contained in the air passing through the membrane will be filtered out. One such system is shown in Figure 14.4. The membrane is removed from the filter holder and placed on top of an agar plate, incubated, and the micro-organisms that grow into colonies counted.

A membrane filter with a grid printed on the surface will assist in counting the micro-organisms. Filters made from gelatine can also be used; the gelatine retains moisture, and it has been reported that this assists in preventing death of the micro-organisms by desiccation.

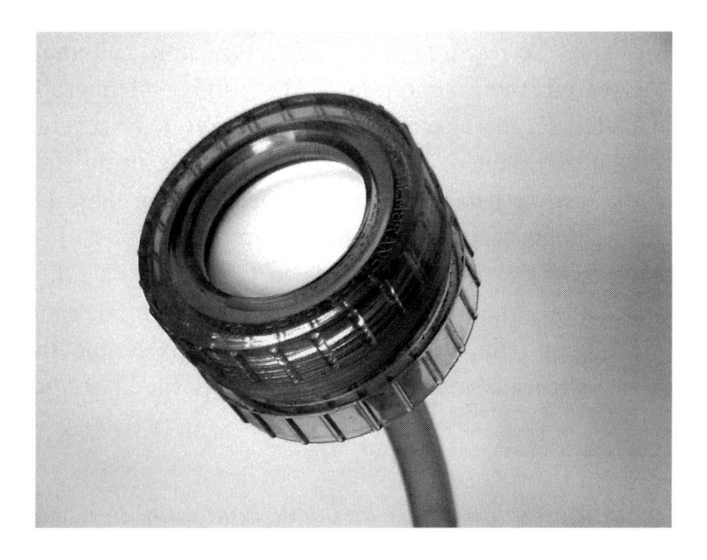

Figure 14.4 Membrane holder with filter

14.2 Microbial Deposition onto Surfaces

14.2.1 Settle plate sampling

In the previous section of this chapter, volumetric microbial sampling of the air in cleanrooms has been described. However, volumetric sampling of airborne micro-organisms is an indirect measurement of the likelihood of micro-organisms depositing on, or into, products manufactured in the cleanroom. The direct method is by settle plate sampling.

As will be discussed in Section 19.2, micro-organisms in the air of occupied cleanrooms are usually found rafted on skin particles. These microbe-carrying particles are, in cleanroom terms, of a substantial size and have an average equivalent particle diameter of between about 10 μm to 30 μm. They can therefore deposit, by gravity, onto surfaces at an average rate of about 1 cm/s.

In settle plate sampling, Petri dishes containing agar medium are opened and exposed for a given period of time, thus allowing microbe-carrying particles to deposit onto them. Petri dishes, 90 mm in diameter (internal area 64 cm^2) are frequently used but in high quality cleanrooms, with their attendant low airborne contamination, larger 140 mm (internal area 154 cm^2) Petri dishes are more appropriate. The number of microbe-carrying particles deposited on the agar surface of the plate over several hours of exposure is then ascertained. Four to five hours is a useful period, as it coincides with the time personnel are in the cleanroom; there is also little loss of micro-organisms caused by desiccation.

Petri dishes must be about two-thirds to three-quarters full of agar to minimise desiccation. The microbial deposition rate can be reported as the number depositing onto the area of a Petri dish in a given time; this rate can also be more scientifically reported as number deposited per hour, per 100 cm^2.

14.2.2 Calculation of the likely airborne contamination

If the exposed area of a product and the time that it is exposed to airborne microbial contamination during manufacture is known, then it is possible to calculate the product's contamination rate. Using the number of microbe-carrying particles deposited on a Petri dish in a given time and proportioning the areas and times of exposure, the contamination rate can be calculated from the following equation:

$$\text{Contamination rate} = \text{Settle plate count x } \frac{\text{area of product}}{\text{area of petri dish}} \text{ x } \frac{\text{time product exposed}}{\text{time settle plates exposed}}$$

Example: A 14 cm Petri dish (154 cm^2 area) is laid close to where containers are filled and the microbial count on the settle plate after four hours of exposure was 3. The number of micro-organisms likely to deposit into the container of a neck area of 1 cm^2, when they are open during filling, for an average of 10 minutes is therefore:

$$3 \times \frac{1}{154} \times \frac{10}{60 \times 4} = 0.0008 \text{ (8 containers in 10 000)}$$

14.3 Microbial Surface Sampling

Several methods are available for microbial surface sampling, but two are commonly used in cleanrooms. These are contact sampling and swabbing.

14.3.1 Contact surface sampling

Contact plates and strips are used when the cleanroom surface to be sampled is relatively flat. If plates are used, then RODAC (Replicate Organisms Detection And Counting) dishes of the type shown in Figure 14.5 are used. These dishes are often 55 mm in diameter with the inner dish covered by a lid resting on a lip. Pouring 15.5 ml to 16 ml of agar medium into the central chamber fills it and gives an agar meniscus that stands proud of the rim.

The agar is rolled over the cleanroom surface to be sampled. Micro-organisms will stick to the agar and when the dish is incubated for a suitable time and temperature, the micro-organisms will grow into colonies that can be counted. When disinfectants are used there is likely to be a residue left on the surface that is sampled. The residue may stop the growth of micro-organisms and chemicals that neutralise the action of disinfectants should be incorporated into the agar medium to prevent this.

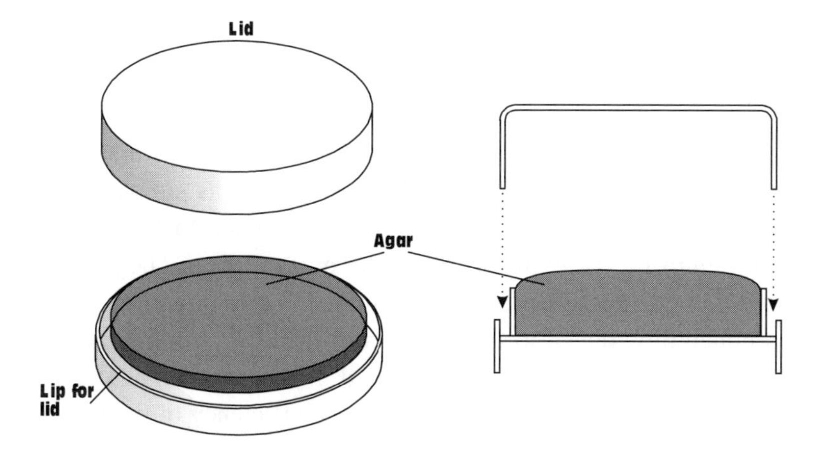

Figure 14.5 Contact plate

Agar contact strips of the type shown in Figure 14.6 are also used to sample surfaces. These strips are removed from their container and applied to the surface to be sampled. The micro-organisms stick to the agar surface and the number ascertained by incubation and counting the colonies that grow.

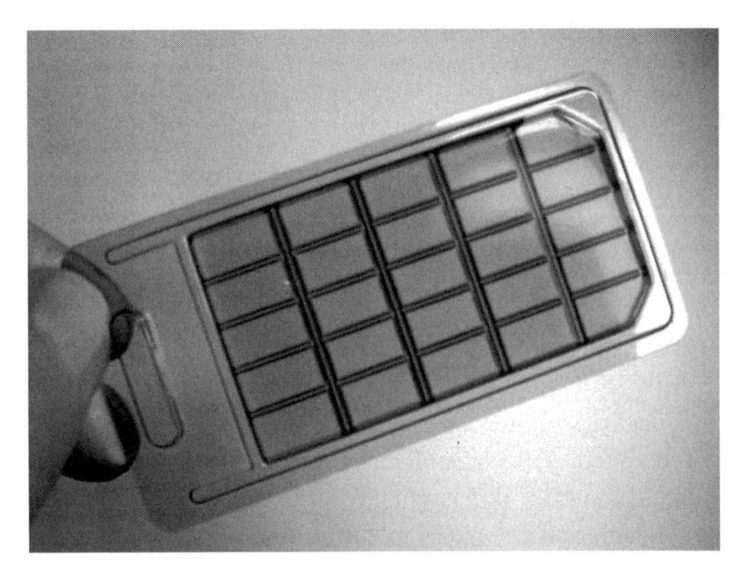

Figure 14.6 Contact strip

14.3.2 Swabbing

To sample uneven surfaces, a commonly used method is the application of a bud swab made from a material such as cotton. At its simplest, a sterile swab is randomly rubbed over the cleanroom surface to be sampled (as shown in Figure 14.7) and then rubbed over an agar plate. The plate is then incubated and the microbial count determined. To improve the efficiency and reproducibility, the swab should be dampened with a sterile liquid such as saline and a known surface area sampled. Methods, such as shaking the swab in liquid can also be used to increase the efficiency of the removal of micro-organisms from the swab.

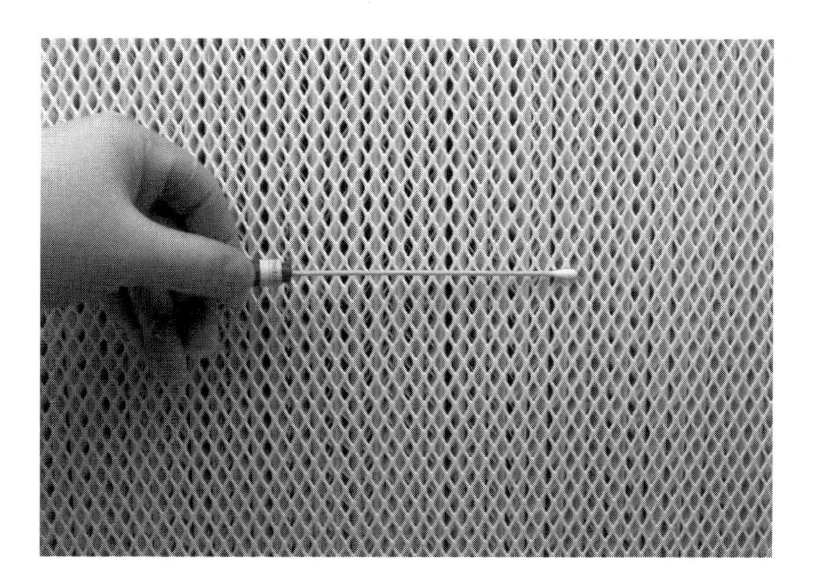

Figure 14.7 Swabbing with a bud swab

14.4 Personnel sampling

Personnel are the primary source of micro-organisms in a cleanroom, and it may be necessary to monitor them to ensure that there is no unusually high dispensers of micro-organisms working within the cleanroom. It may also be necessary, when unusually high concentrations of micro-organisms are found in the air, surfaces, or within the product, to find the person who is the source. The methods commonly used are:

- Finger dabs. The person's fingers tips, or their gloved hand, is pressed or wiped on an agar plate and the number of micro-organisms ascertained.
- Contact plates or strips. The person's garments are sampled by pressing the plate or strip onto their clothing. This is best done as they come out of the cleanroom.
- Body box. If a person wearing normal indoor clothing exercises within a body box their dispersion rate of airborne micro-organisms can be ascertained. (See Section 19.6.1.)

Acknowledgements

Figure 14.2 is reproduced by permission of International pbi. Figure 14.3 is reproduced by permission of Biotest.

15

Operating a Cleanroom: Contamination Control

The initial chapters of this book describe how a cleanroom is designed and constructed. Further chapters describe the tests required to ascertain that a cleanroom performed correctly when new, and throughout its life. In the final seven chapters I shall discuss how cleanrooms should be operated to minimise the risk of contamination. This chapter introduces the topic by considering the sources and routes of contamination within a cleanroom and how to control these.

To be able to control contamination in a cleanroom it is first of all necessary to assess the various risks. A number of systems exist for assessing risk during manufacturing, such as *Fault Tree Analysis (FTA)* and *Failure Mode and Effect Analysis (FMEA)*.

These systems appear to have been written for electrical and mechanical systems but can be applied to all types of risks. Those who are expert in working with such systems will be able to apply them to contamination risks. However, the majority of cleanroom users will more easily understand the *Hazard Analysis and Critical Control Point (HACCP)* system. This was devised, and is now used extensively, to prevent contamination in the food production industry. However, the system needs some reinterpretation and modification for application to cleanrooms in general.

HACCP has a seven-step approach, but this requires some additions and re-arrangement to make it more understandable to the cleanroom user. I suggest the following system:

1. Identify the sources of contamination in the cleanroom. Construct a risk diagram, or diagrams, to show these sources and their routes of contamination.
2. Assess the importance of these sources and whether, or not, they are hazards that need to be controlled.
3. Identify methods that can be used to control these hazards.
4. Determine valid sampling methods to monitor either the hazards, or their control methods, or both.
5. Establish a monitoring schedule with 'alert' and 'action' levels and corrective measures to be taken, where appropriate, when these levels are exceeded.
6. Verify that the contamination control system is working effectively by reviewing the product rejection rate, sampling results and control methods and, where appropriate, modifying them.
7. Establish and maintain appropriate documentation.
8. Train the staff.

15.1 Step 1: Identification of Sources and Routes of Contamination

15.1.1 Sources of contamination

Examples of sources of contamination in a cleanroom are as follows:

- dirty areas adjacent to the cleanroom
- unfiltered air supply
- room air
- surfaces
- people
- machines, as they work

- raw materials
- containers
- packaging.

Areas adjacent to the cleanroom are likely to be less-clean than the production cleanroom; the material airlock and clothing-change areas will be contaminated by the activities going on in these areas, and the contamination in the outside corridors and service plenums may not be controlled. The air supplied to a room, if not correctly filtered, is a source of contamination. Room air is also a source if it contains contamination dispersed into it from other sources, such as people and machines.

The floor, walls, ceiling and other surfaces in the cleanroom are examples of surface sources, their contamination being mostly derived from personnel touching them, or contamination depositing from the air. These surfaces can also be sources of contamination if poor quality constructional components are used, which break up and disperse fibres, wood chips, plaster etc.

Cleanroom clothing, gloves and masks are other surfaces that are contaminated either by the people wearing them or by other cleanroom surfaces. Personnel within the cleanroom can disperse contamination from the skin, mouth and clothing. This contamination can be transferred to the product through the air, or by contact with their hands or clothing.

Machines are another source, as they can generate contamination by the movement of their constituent parts, or by generation by thermal, electrical or other means. Raw materials, containers and packaging that are brought in, or piped into the cleanroom, may be contaminated and should be considered as sources.

15.1.2 Airborne and contact routes of transfer

As well as identifying the sources of contamination in a cleanroom, the routes of transfer must be considered. The two main routes are airborne and contact.

Contamination can be dispersed into the air from all the main sources and transferred to the product. If the particles are small they can float off to other parts of the cleanroom. However, if they are large, like fibres, chips or cuttings they will remain within a short distance from where they were generated, and fall directly into, or on to, the product.

Contact routes of contamination occur when machines, containers, packaging, raw materials, gloves, clothes, etc. come directly into contact with the product. Contact contamination can occur in several ways; one example is when personnel handle a product and the contamination on their gloves is transferred onto the product and another is when the product comes into contact with dirty containers or packaging.

Using information of the type discussed in this and the previous section, the sources and routes of transfer can be ascertained and a risk diagram constructed for any cleanroom.

15.1.3 Construction of a risk diagram

Construction of a 'risk diagram' is a good method of understanding how contamination arises from sources and then reaches the product. The way in which a product is contaminated is often poorly understood but, by constructing a risk diagram, a greater understanding will follow. The risk diagram should show possible sources of contamination, their main routes of transfer, and methods of controlling this transfer. It may be necessary to construct several diagrams where the process is complex, or where it is necessary to control different contaminants, e.g. particles, microbe-carrying particles and molecular contamination.

Figure 15.1 is an example of a risk diagram showing the main sources of bacterial and particle contamination in a typical cleanroom. It also includes the main routes of transfer of contamination and the means of controlling it. The transfer of contamination around the room can be very complicated as, in theory, everything in the cleanroom can be contaminated by everything else. However, in practice, it should only be necessary to consider the major ones. It is interesting to note the central role of air, which receives and transports the many types of contaminants in a cleanroom.

The manufacturing process has been excluded from Figure 15.1. This is shown separately in Figure 15.2.

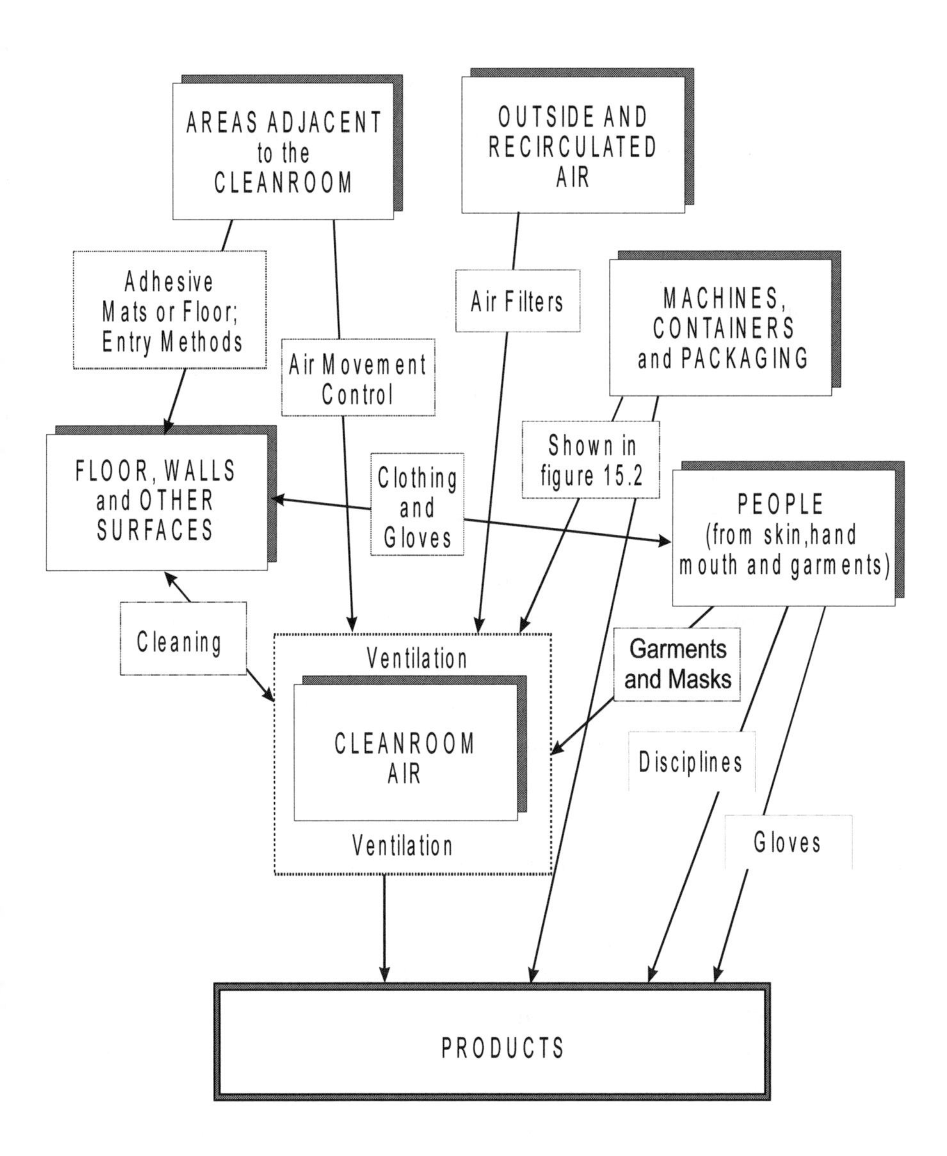

Figure 15.1 Sources and routes of particle and microbial contamination in a cleanroom along with preventative measures

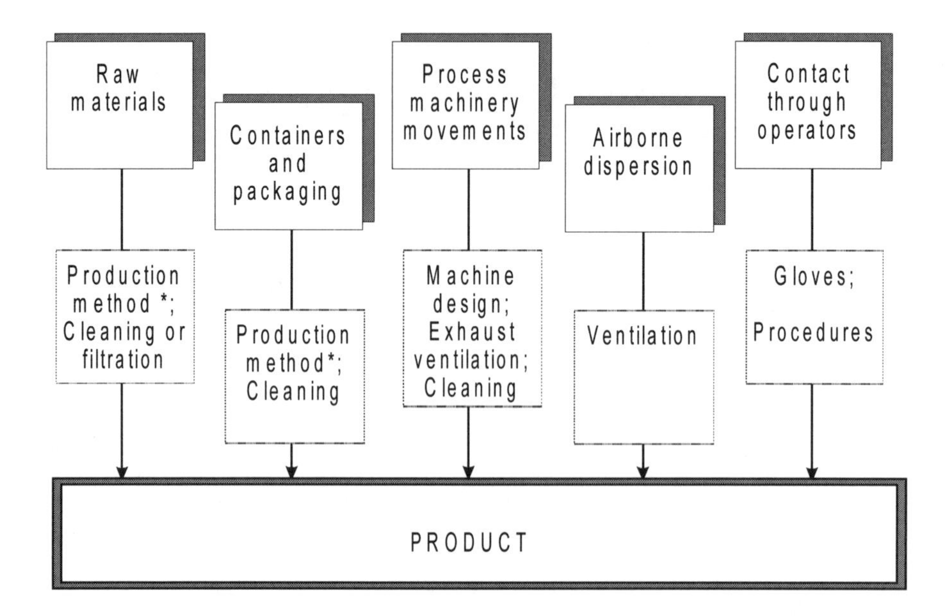

Figure 15.2 Sources and routes of control associated with process machinery. * contamination of the raw materials, containers and packaging can be controlled by producing them in suitably clean conditions

15.2 Step 2: Assessment of the Importance of Hazards

When all possible sources of contamination in the cleanroom, and their routes of transmission, have been identified, the next task is to carry out a risk assessment. This is also called hazard or risk analysis. It ascertains what sources of contamination are important, i.e. if they are a hazard and their relative importance, or degree of risk.

It is often difficult to determine which contamination sources are the most hazardous. This is especially difficult if the cleanroom is new and not yet operational, as few useful monitoring results will have been collected. However lack of monitoring results should not prevent a preliminary assessment being made, as it will be possible at a later stage (Step 6) to return to these tentative conclusions for a reappraisal and, if necessary, make changes.

To determine the likely importance of a hazard, I suggest the following method. Firstly, a set of variables known as risk factors should be determined. These are:

- the amount of contamination on, or in, the source that is available for transfer (risk factor A);
- the ease by which the contamination is dispersed or transferred (risk factor B);
- the proximity of the source to the critical point where the product is exposed (risk factor C);
- how easily the contamination can pass through the control method (risk factor D).

Table 15.1 shows the risk factors and score values that can be used to assess the overall risk rating, or hazard, of each individual source. Each of these factors (A to D) should be assessed and given a score of 0 to 2.

Table 15.1 Risk factors for assessing hazards

Amount of contamination on, or in, a source (A)	Ease of dispersion, or transfer (B)	Proximity from critical area (C)	Penetration through control method (D)
0 = nil	0 = nil	0 = outside corridor	0 = barrier protection
0.5 = very low	0.5 = very low	0.5 = air lock	0.5 = very good control
1 = low	1 = low	1 = periphery of cleanroom	1 = good control
1.5 = medium	1.5 = medium	1.5 = general area of cleanroom	1.5 = some control
2 = high	2 = high	2 = critical area	2 = no control

Using Equation (15.1) the four scores should be multiplied together to obtain a risk rating. This will have a value of 0 to 16.

$$\text{Risk rating} = \text{A} \times \text{B} \times \text{C} \times \text{D} \qquad (15.1)$$

A risk rating can therefore be obtained for each contamination source and this rating can be used to determine the importance of each source and whether it is a hazard to the product. If required, the risk rating can assigned a 'low', 'medium' or 'high' category. For example, a risk rating of less than 4 can be considered as 'low', between 4 and 12 as 'medium' and higher that 12 'high'. Experience with the system will help develop a useable system. This risk rating can then be used to help determine how much effort should be put into controlling each source. However, it should be appreciated that this method should only be used to *assist* in assessing the risks. The quality of the information available as input and the inexact nature of the mathematical model means that it cannot give exact predictions.

Two examples of a risk assessment will demonstrate the general method.

Example 1: A risk assessment is required to answer the question 'how great a hazard are cleanroom walls'. Firstly, the 'amount of contamination' factor (A) should be assessed. As the amount of contamination on the walls is 'low', a score of 1 could be given. The 'ease of dispersion or transfer' (B) is likely to be 'very low' and given a score of 0.5. As the wall is at the periphery of the room, a value of 1 is given to the 'proximity' score (C). A score of 1 might be an appropriate score for the 'control of the source' (D) if the wall was cleaned frequently, 1.5 if it was cleaned irregularly and 2 if it was never cleaned. Thus, the overall hazard assessment score of between 0.5 and 1 would be obtained. This demonstrates that walls are not an important hazard.

Example 2: The hands of a person handling a product are considered. Maximum scores of 2 and 2 could be given for the 'amount of contamination' (A) and 'the ease of dispersion, or transfer' (B), as hands have very large amounts of particles, bacteria and salts and these are easily transferred when personnel handle the product. A maximum score of 2 could also be assigned to the 'proximity from the critical area'. The overall hazard assessment score is now dependent on how the hand contamination is controlled. If no gloves are worn, a hazard score close to the maximum of 16 can be calculated from Equation (15.1). If gloves were worn, then depending on how likely they were to be punctured, an overall hazard score of about 8 would be obtained. The use of double gloves, or gauntlets in an isolator, would give either very good control, or barrier protection, this would reduce the overall hazard score to close to 0. It can be seen from this example that hands are a high potential hazard and their control is important.

15.3 Step 3: Identification of Methods to Control Hazards

When all the contamination hazards in the cleanroom have been identified and their degree of risk assessed, it is then necessary to review the methods available to control them. The importance of obtaining an effective control method should be related to the above risk assessment; the greater the risk, the more effective the control method should be. It is also necessary to show that the control method is effective. If it is not then either a more effective control method should be adopted or the control method applied to a different point or place. Figures 15.1 and 15.2 show methods that can be used to control the routes of spread of contamination. These are:

1. HEPA or ULPA air filters can be used to prevent any contaminants entering with the supply air. However, unfiltered air can pass through holes in damaged filters, or by-pass the filter owing to poor filter housing construction.
2. Airborne contamination from areas outside the cleanroom, e.g. outside corridors and service plenums, can be prevented from entering the cleanroom by ensuring that the air moves from the cleanroom outwards, i.e. from clean to less-clean. Air locks and, or, a cascade flow of air through the doorways will ensure this. The use of adhesive cleanroom mats and flooring, as well as the removal, or covering, of dirty

outdoor shoes prevents surface contamination being transferred into the cleanroom.

3. Although cleanroom air is a transfer route, it is also a source. Such airborne sources of contamination can be reduced by the use of a conventional ventilation system to dilute it, a unidirectional ventilation system to sweep it away, or an isolator or minienvironment to provide a barrier.
4. The possibility of transfer of contamination from the floors, walls and ceiling is minimised by cleaning, and any contamination that becomes airborne is controlled by ventilation.
5. People disperse contamination from their mouth, hair, clothing and skin. Cleanroom garments and gloves will minimise this dispersion and contamination that cannot be controlled (as well as that produced by their clothing) can be minimised by the ventilation system.
6. Contamination from machines can be minimised by the design of the machine, or by the use of exhaust air systems to draw the contamination away. Cleaning can control dirt on the machine.
7. Raw materials used to make products, or from which products are assembled, as well as containers and packaging, should be made from materials that do not generate contamination. They should also be manufactured in an environment that ensures that they have minimal concentrations of contamination on, or within, them. They should be correctly wrapped to ensure that they are not contaminated during delivery and that when the packaging is removed, on entry, contamination does not occur. Materials that are not sufficiently clean will require to be cleaned or, if fluid, filtered.

15.4 Step 4: Sampling Methods to Monitor Hazards and Control Methods

It will now be necessary to set limits to ensure that contamination of the manufacturing process is kept under control. If air is taken as an example, then there are well-established methods of measuring particles and microorganisms, and standards such as ISO 14644-1 should be used to set limits. However, if personnel handling the product cause the hazard, and the control measure is the wearing of gloves, monitoring could be by inspecting for punctures and tears in the gloves, or measurement of particles or micro-organisms on the surfaces.

The methods used to monitor hazards within a cleanroom and the frequency of sampling are discussed in previous chapters. Given in Table 15.2 are some well-known cleanroom hazards, their routes of transfer and control, and how to monitor them. Also given in the table is the section of this book where further information may be found.

Table 15.2 Sources, routes of transfer and control and monitoring methods used in cleanrooms.

Hazard	Route	Control method	Monitoring methods	Section reference
Supply air	airborne	air filters	filter integrity test	chapter 12
Areas adjacent to the cleanroom	airborne	overpressure; air movement control	room pressure differential	10.2; 11.1
	contact	cleanroom mats	mat inspection	17.2.1
Various airborne dispersions	airborne	ventilation	air supply rate or velocity	10.1
			counts of airborne particles	chapter 13
			counts of airborne micro-organisms	14.1
			control of airflow	11.2
Floors, walls and other surfaces	contact	cleaning (and, where required, disinfection)	surface counting of particles,	21.6
			and micro-organisms	14.3
People	airborne	cleanroom garments	surface counts; inspection for tears; particle penetration testing	19.6

	contact	gloves	inspection for punctures	20.2.4
			surface contamination counts	20.2.4
Machines	airborne	ventilation	air extract rates and airflow patterns	10.1, 11.2
	contact	design of machine;	—	—
		cleaning or disinfection	surface contamination	21.6
Raw materials	mainly contact	control of manufacturing of raw materials	particle and bacterial counts within, or on, the materials.	not discussed
		cleaning if solid, or filtration if fluids	filtration systems	not discussed
		sterilisation	sterilisation system	not discussed
Containers and packaging	mainly contact	control of their composition and manufacturing environment	particle and microbial counts on surface	not discussed
		sterilisation	sterilisation system	not discussed

Step 4 of the contamination control system outlined in Section 15.1, requires a '*valid* sampling method'. The term 'validate' can be defined as 'ensuring that something is fit for the purpose, or works well in the situation in which it is being used'. In terms of monitoring, the following may require to be demonstrated:

- collection efficiency of sampling instruments;
- calibration of the instruments;
- determination that the hazard is of sufficient importance to need to be monitored;
- determination that the sampling method used is the best available for *directly* measuring the hazard, or its control method.

The last two requirements are not always easy to determine but, if correctly done, they will ensure that the monitoring effort is not wasted.

15.5 Step 5: Establishing a Monitoring Schedule with Alert and Action Levels

Some monitoring systems are continuous, as is the case with particle counting in high quality cleanrooms, but on the other hand, some inconsequential contamination sources, such as the ceiling, are not monitored. The frequency of monitoring will have to be determined for each hazard or control method, for each individual cleanroom. This should be set up with due regard to the importance of the hazard; the higher the risk, the more frequent the sampling should be.

It is also necessary to decide what corrective actions should be taken when the monitoring results show that the hazard is not under control. A useful approach here is to set 'alert' and 'action' conditions; these are also called 'warning' and 'alarm' levels. In a cleanroom, it will be normal to consider only upper limits and ignore the lower ones, as low contamination levels are not a hazard. The 'alert' level should be set to indicate that the contamination concentrations are higher than might be expected, but are still under control. Nothing will normally be done if the 'alert' level is exceeded, as this is a warning to be on the alert for future problems. However, several 'alerts' in a relatively short time might suggest that action is required. The 'action' level should be set such that when it is exceeded there should be an investigation. An assessment should be made as to whether it is a spurious result caused by natural variation, a mistake in the collection of the results, or a real result. For those results that are considered 'real', there should be an investigation by a method that has been set down; this should assess whether or not the result is acceptable and, if not, what action is required to bring the situation under control.

Analysing the monitoring results and setting 'alert' and 'action' levels is quite a complicated subject if a statistical approach is used. Knowledge of statistical techniques, especially the use of trend analysis and Shewhart and CUSUM charts is required; a discussion of these is outside the scope of this book. However, a simple approach can be taken by choosing appropriate numbers from the available data, or seeking advice from the suppliers of the instruments used to monitor the contamination.

15.6 Step 6: Verification and Reappraisal of the System

A method must now be set in place to check that the system has been correctly implemented. Its usefulness might be indicated by the rejection rate of the product; as long as this is satisfactory then the system could be considered to be working well. However, it is also possible at this time to attempt to reduce the rejection rate by introducing a further control method.

Verification that the system is working well can also be carried out by measurement of the particle, or microbial, levels in samples of the final product. Simulation of the process, e.g. filling containers with microbiological medium and ascertaining the microbial contamination, is a method that is useful in some circumstances. It is also possible to verify the effectiveness of the control measures by inspection and assessment of the monitoring results.

We can now reassess the following:

1. the relative importance of the hazards
2. the necessity and the methods for controlling the hazards
3. the effectiveness of the control methods
4. the correctness of the monitoring schedule
5. whether the 'action' and 'alert' levels should be lowered or raised.

15.7 Step 7: Documentation

An effective contamination control system will document (1) the methods described in the preceding steps of this chapter, (2) the monitoring procedures, and (3) results from the monitoring. The first two groups should be regularly updated to incorporate changes.

Regular reports should be issued of an analysis of the monitoring results and any deviations from the expected results. When 'action' levels are exceeded these should be reported. The actions taken to correct the deviations, or the explanations as to why no action was necessary, should also be documented. 'Alert' levels can also be reported, particularly those with a multiple or unusual occurrence.

15.8 Step 8: Staff Training

All efforts to control contamination will fail if the personnel working in the cleanroom do not understand how the room works, and how they should conduct themselves within the cleanroom to minimise contamination. They should be trained in these aspects of contamination, both when they first arrive at the cleanroom and at regular intervals throughout their careers. Suitable items for a syllabus can be selected from the index of this book.

16

Cleanroom Disciplines

Cleanroom personnel are a important source of cleanroom contamination. Almost all micro-organisms found in a cleanroom come from personnel, and they are also a major source of particles and fibres. It is therefore necessary to ensure the minimum of contamination is generated and transferred by personnel activities. By observing certain disciplines, contamination of the product can be minimised. These are discussed in this chapter.

When a cleanroom is about to be opened, management is faced with the task of employing people to work in the room, and determining what disciplines personnel (including maintenance and service technicians) should adhere to within the cleanroom. It is hoped that this chapter will assist in this task.

It should be noted that products manufactured in a cleanroom vary in their sensitivity to contamination, and cleanroom disciplines should reflect this. The information given in this chapter are options from which the user can choose methods that best reflect the degree of risk associated with their cleanroom.

16.1 People Allowed into Cleanrooms

People can, when walking, produce about 1 000 000 particles ≥ 0.5 μm and several thousand microbe-carrying particles per minute. The more people, the higher the dispersion within the cleanroom. It is therefore important that the minimum of people, i.e. only the essential personnel are allowed into cleanrooms, and management should ensure that this is so.

Because many contamination problems are caused by lack of knowledge, only people trained to work in a cleanroom should be allowed within the cleanroom. Personnel should therefore be formally trained in the various aspects of contamination control. Visitors should be discouraged and only allowed in under the control of a supervisor; if a cleanroom is designed with windows for visitors to look into the cleanroom, this will usually suffice. Special care should be taken with service and maintenance technicians, and their tools and materials; this is discussed at the end of this chapter.

People who enter the cleanroom should not disperse significantly greater amounts of contamination than the normal population. Given below are examples of conditions that can cause more contamination than normal, and may therefore be unacceptable. Acceptability will depend on the risk, e.g. whether micro-organisms are a hazard, and whether the product is highly susceptible to contamination or not. It will therefore be up to management to decide which conditions are important.

The following suggestions contain criteria that can discriminate against some personnel. It should be ensured that any discrimination is neither illegal nor unfair. The list also contains a number of temporary conditions. These are included as they may be a reason for temporarily assigning personnel to a job outside the cleanroom.

- Skin conditions where unusually large amounts of skin cells are dispersed, such as dermatitis, sunburn or bad dandruff.
- Respiratory conditions such as coughing or sneezing caused by colds, flu or chronic lung disease.
- In a biocleanroom, it may be necessary to screen personnel for the carriage of micro-organisms that could grow in the product and cause spoilage or disease. Their suitability for work in a cleanroom should be considered with respect to the susceptibility of the product to specific types of microbial growth.
- People with allergic conditions, which cause sneezing, itching, scratching, or a running nose, may not be suitable for employment in a cleanroom. Sufferers from hay fever are likely to find relief in a cleanroom because the air filtration system will filter out the allergens responsible. Some people may be allergic to materials used in the cleanroom, such as (a) garments made from polyester, (b) plastic or latex gloves, (c) chemicals such as acids, solvents, cleaning agents and dis-

infectants, and (d) products manufactured in the room, e.g. antibiotics and hormones.

Depending on the contamination risk within the cleanroom, some or all of the following suggestions should be brought to the attention of the staff so that contamination within the room may be minimised:

- Personnel should have a good level of personal hygiene. They should shower regularly and keep dandruff at bay. They should wash their hair after a haircut to prevent hair landing on the product. In the case of dry skin, they should use skin lotion to replace skin oil that is lacking; this should reduce dispersion.
- Materials such as cosmetics, talcum powder, hair sprays, nail polish, or similar materials are not normally allowed in a cleanrooms. Anything added on to the body should generally be considered a contaminant. Cosmetics are a particular problem in semiconductor manufacturing as they contain a large amount of inorganic ions such as titanium, iron, aluminium, calcium, barium, sodium and magnesium. In the photographic industry, iron and iodine ions give problems. Other industries, which do not have a problem with specific chemicals, may still experience problems as each application will deposit large numbers of particles (up to 10^9 for particles ≥ 0.5 μm) on the skin. Some of these will detach in the cleanroom.
- Watches and jewellery are normally not allowed in a cleanroom. If jewellery is allowed, it must be under the clothing and gloves. Rings can puncture gloves and harbour contamination under them. Personnel may be reluctant, for sentimental reasons, to remove their wedding or engagement rings. They may be allowed to keep them on if the skin under the rings, as well as the rings, is washed. Where the rings are liable to puncture the glove they should be taped over.
- Smokers are said to produce more particles from their mouth than the normal population and outgas chemicals from their body. It may be necessary to ensure that they have not smoked for several hours before entering the cleanroom. It has been reported that taking a drink of water before entering the cleanroom reduces the number of particles given off from the mouth.

16.2 Personal Items Not Allowed into the Cleanroom.

As a general rule, nothing should be allowed into the cleanroom that is not required for production within the room. However, it is up to the management of the cleanroom to decide what items could cause contamination of the product. Items that should be considered for inclusion in a list of prohibited items are:

- food, drink, sweets and chewing gum
- cans or bottles
- smoking materials
- radios, CD players, Walkmans, cell phones, pagers, etc.
- newspapers, magazines, books and paper handkerchiefs
- pencils and erasers
- wallets, purses and other similar items.

Given in Section 18.2 of this book is a list of materials that may be required for manufacturing, and be sources of contamination. Some of the items from that list may be added to the above list.

16.3 Disciplines within the Cleanroom

Within a cleanroom, many rules-of-conduct must be followed to ensure that products are not contaminated. The management must produce a set of written procedures suitable for their room. It may be useful to have these 'does and don'ts' posted in the change or production area. Commonly used procedures that may be adopted are given below. These procedures do not consider the choice of cleanroom garments, masks, gloves and similar clothing items. Information about items of attire is given in Chapter 19.

16.3.1 Air transfer

To ensure that air is not transferred from an area of high contamination to one of lower contamination (e.g. the outside corridor to the production room) the following disciplines should be adhered to:

1. Personnel must always come in and out of the cleanroom through change areas. The change area is used not only to change clothing, but as a buffer zone between the outer dirty corridor and the inner clean production area. Personnel should not use any entrance, such as an emergency exit, which leads directly from the production area to the corridor; this will allow contamination to enter directly into the cleanroom, and their garments may also become contaminated.
2. Doors should not be left open. If they are, air will be transferred between the two adjoining areas because of general air turbulence as well as air transfer caused by a temperature difference between the two areas (Figure 16.1).

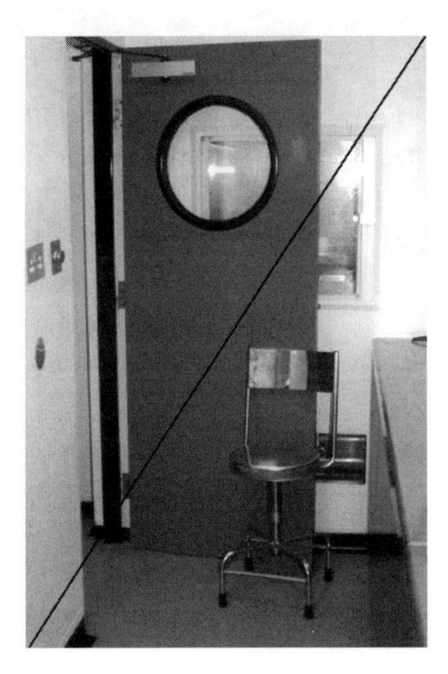

Figure 16.1 Doors should not be left open

3. Doors should not be opened or closed quickly, or air will be pumped from one area to the other.
4. Doors usually open inwards into the production room and are held shut by the higher pressure. However, to aid the movement of personnel who are

carrying materials, some doors open outwards. Doors should then be fitted with door-closing devices to ensure that the doors are kept closed, and shut slowly to reduce the air transfer (Figure 16.3). Doors without handles will assist in preventing contamination of gloves.

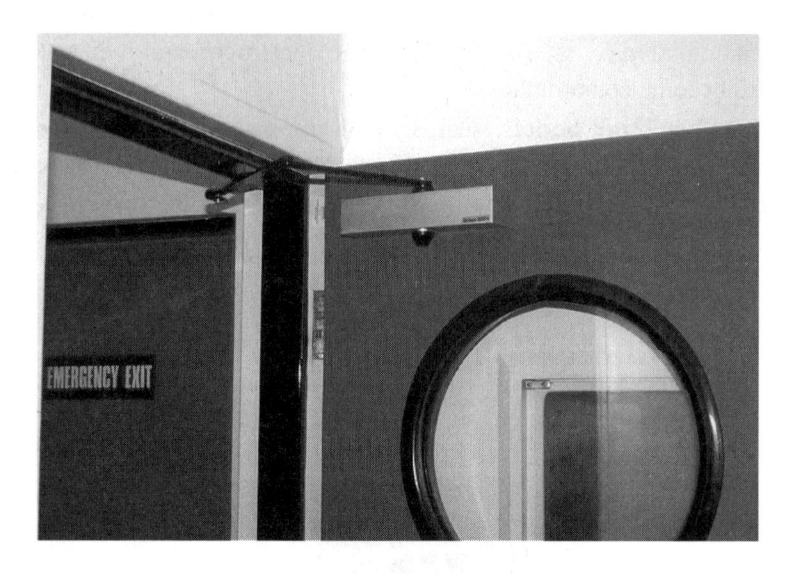

16.2 Door closing device may be used

5. When passing through the doors in an airlock, personnel should ensure the first door is closed before going through the next one. Electrical interlocks between entry and exit doors achieve this, but care must be taken to ensure that there is no danger in the case of fire. Indicator lights, which show if the doors are shut, are also used. Pass-through hatches should be used in a similar way.

16.3.2 Personnel behaviour

The following suggestions should be considered to ensure that personnel do not contribute to the contamination within the room:

1. Silly behaviour should not be allowed. The generation of contamination is proportional to *activity* (Figure 16.3). A motionless person can generate

about 100 000 particles ≥ 0.5 μm/min. A person with head, arms and body moving can generate about 1 000 000 particles ≥ 0.5 μm/min. A person who is walking can generate about 5 000 000 particles ≥ 0.5 μm/min.

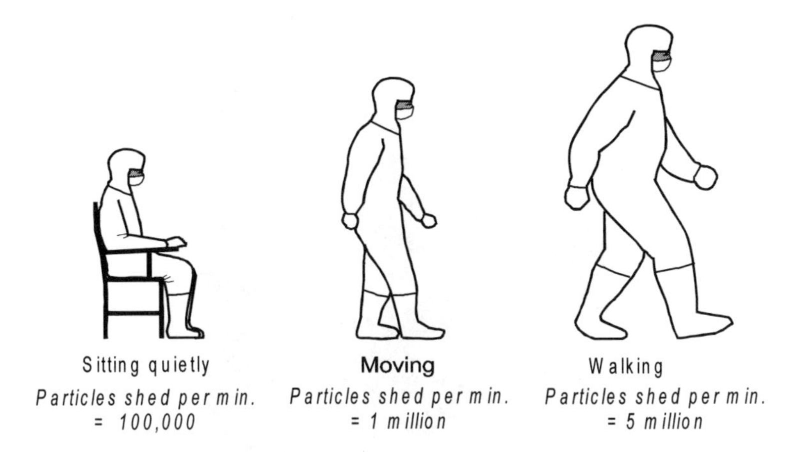

Figure 16.3 Particle dispersion in relation to movement

2. Personnel should position themselves correctly with respect to the product, so that contamination does not land on it (Figure 16.4). They should not lean over the product in such a way that particles, fibres or microbe-carrying particles, fall from personnel onto the product. If personnel are working in a flow of unidirectional air, they should make sure that they are not between the product and the source of the clean air, i.e. the air filter. If they are, a shower of particles could deposit on the product. Methods of working should be pre-planned to minimise this type of contamination.
3. Consideration must be given as to how products are moved or manipulated. 'No-touch' techniques should be devised to prevent contamination getting from the gloved hand onto the product. Although gloves are worn in cleanrooms, they are still likely to be a source of contamination (although a reduced one). An example of this 'no touch' technique is the use of long forceps rather than hands to grip materials (Figure 16.5).

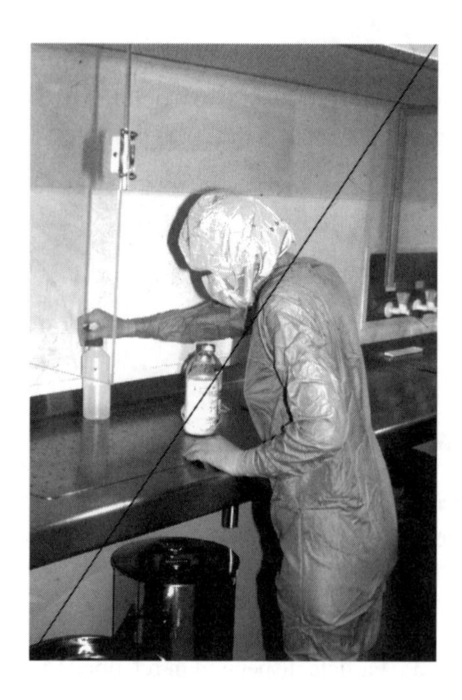

Figure 16.4 Do not lean over and contaminate the product

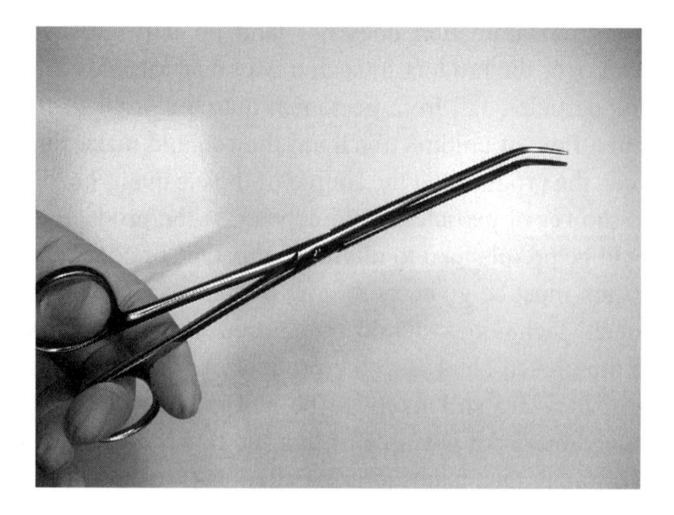

Figure 16.5 Forceps reduce contact contamination

Each cleanroom should have its own 'no-touch' rules to ensure that the product is not contaminated. Shown in Figures 16.6–16.9 are examples of how silicon wafers can be handled in semiconductor areas. These photographs were staged, as it would not be normal practice in a microfabrication facility to handle a silicon wafer except by a vacuum wand, or by robotic means. Figure 16.6 shows the wafer being held by the ungloved hand with the thumb touching the surface.

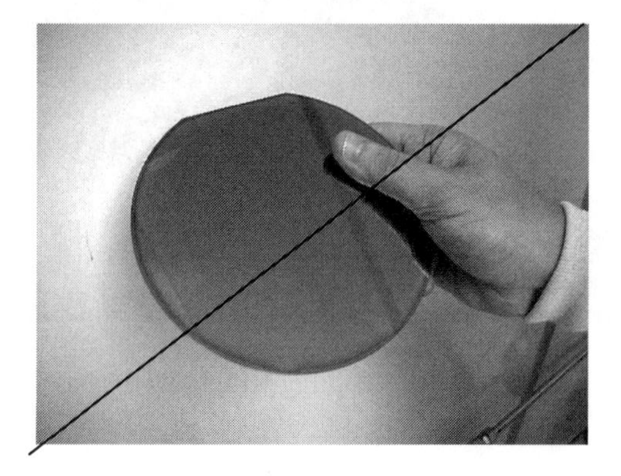

Figure 16.6 Handling with no gloves

Oil and skin particles would contaminate the wafer with catastrophic results. If the wafer is held around the edge of the wafer (Figure 16.7) then contamination is reduced, but can still get onto the surface.

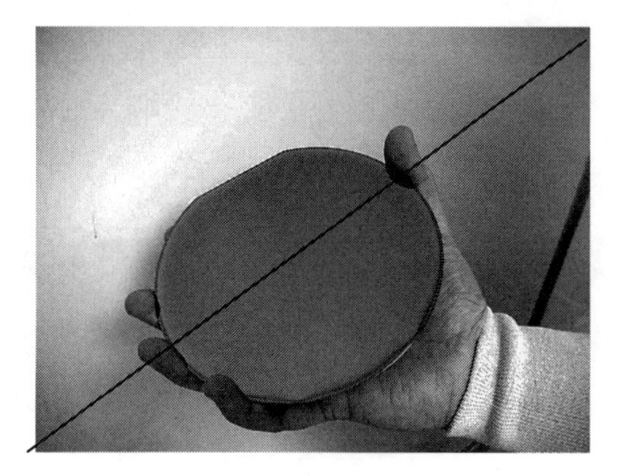

Figure 16.7 Handling at edge without gloves

Use of a glove (Figure 16.8) will reduce contamination yet further, and this technique is still used where the line widths are large and a lower yield acceptable.

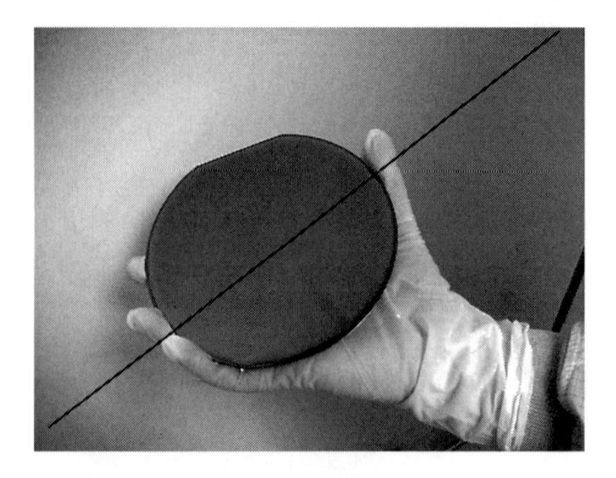

Figure 16.8 Handling with gloved hand

In semiconductor facilities, wafers will be handled with a vacuum wand which attaches itself to the back of the wafer (Figure 16.9). Robotic manipulation can also minimise contamination.

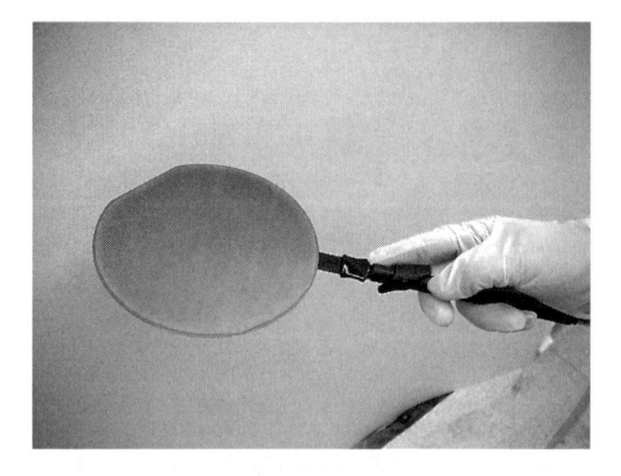

Figure 16.9 Handling with vacuum wand

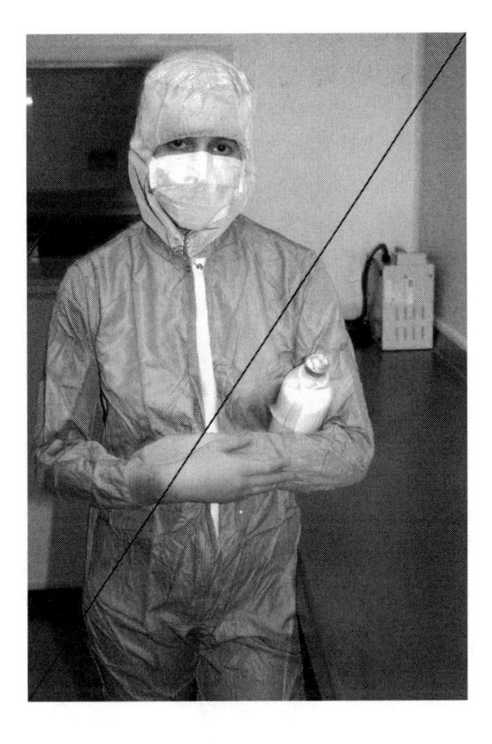

Figure 16.10 Do not support materials next to the body

4. Personnel should not support material against their body (Figure 16.10). Although they will be wearing cleanroom clothing, which is much cleaner than indoor or factory clothing, it is not contamination free. Particles, fibres and micro-organisms can be transferred onto the items carried.

5. Personnel should not talk when working over the product, or spittle from the mouth will pass round the imperfect seal between the mask and the skin and contaminate the product (Figure 16.11). Talking, coughing or sneezing can release contamination from the mask surface. If personnel cough or sneeze, they must turn their head away from the product. Masks are often replaced after sneezing. Masks must not be worn below the nose but over the nose as large particles can be released from the nose when snorting.

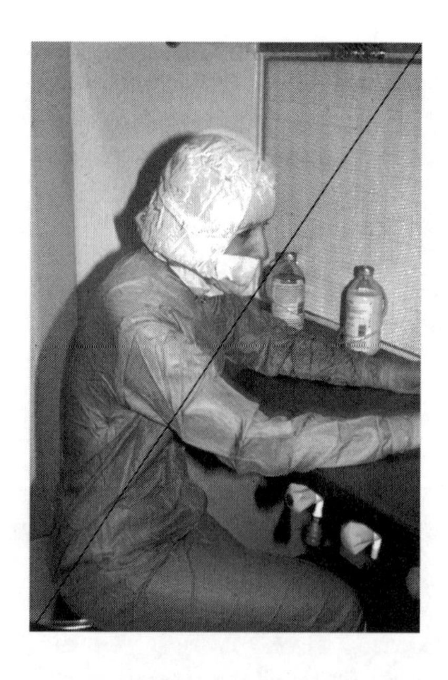

Figure 16.11 Care should be taken to ensure that mask is used correctly

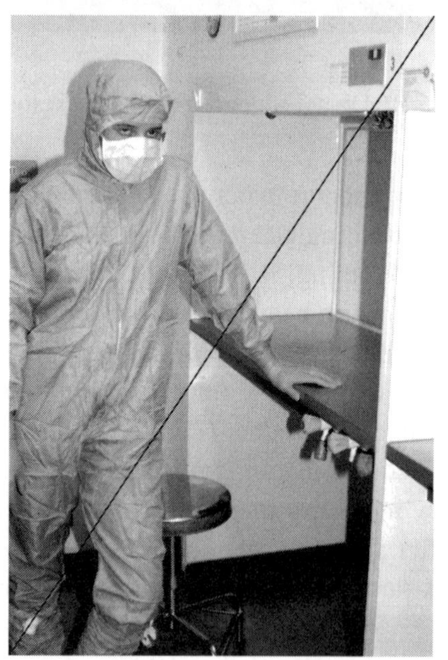

Figure 16.12 Do not touch work surfaces

6. It is generally not good practice for personnel to touch cleanroom surfaces. Although cleanroom surfaces are very much cleaner than those outside the cleanroom, its surfaces, and that of the machinery in the room, will have particles, fibres and bacteria on them. If personnel touch their garments or mask, they also will pick up contamination on their gloves, which may be transferred to the product. Hands grasped together in front of the personnel, in the style of a hospital surgeon, will help to ensure that they do not inadvertently touch surfaces.

7. Personal handkerchiefs should not be brought into cleanrooms (Figure 16.13). These are clearly a major source of contamination and will transfer particles and microbe-carrying particles into the air and onto gloves. Noses should not be blown inside a cleanroom. The change area may be an acceptable alternative.

8. Washing, or disinfection when required, of gloves during use should be considered. Glove washing can be used in cleanrooms where products are handled and there are particular difficulties in keeping gloves clean. For example, in aseptic pharmaceutical production areas, gloved hands are rinsed with a suitable disinfectant (70% ethanol or iso-propanol) at regular intervals and prior to starting a critical operation. Alcohols are particularly useful, as they do not leave a residue on the glove.

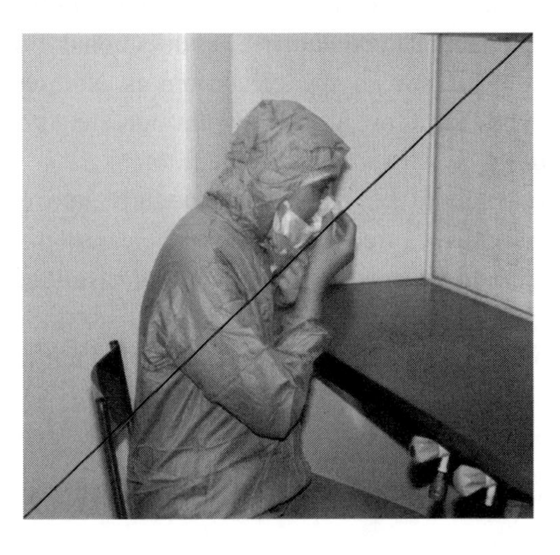

Figure 16.13 Do not use personal handkerchief

16.3.3 Handling materials

The following suggestions, which refer to the materials used in the clean-room, should be considered:

- Cleanroom wipers that have low concentration of contamination should be used. The exact type of wiper that is selected will depend on the financial budget and what is being produced in the cleanroom. It will also be necessary to decide how often a wipe should be used before being discarded. Some additional information is given in Section 20.3.3.
- The movement of materials between the inside and outside of a cleanroom should be minimised. Every time a product moves out of the cleanroom there is a high possibility of it being contaminated in the less-clean area, and this contamination being brought back when it re-enters. It is best to store products in a suitable clean area within the cleanroom, or in an adjoining clean area.
- It is normal to find that great care has been taken to ensure that a product is not contaminated during its manipulation stages. However, after that, it can often be forgotten and left out in the cleanroom to gather dust. Products that are susceptible to contamination should therefore be kept in closed cabinets, containers, unidirectional flow benches, or isolators. If the airflow in the cleanroom is unidirectional, storage racks of the type that allow air to flow through are a good choice. Materials should not be left standing on the floor.
- Waste material should be collected frequently into easily identified containers and removed frequently from the cleanroom.
- Cleanrooms should be correctly cleaned (and disinfected if required). This major topic is discussed in Chapter 21.
- The cleanroom must be kept neat and tidy. If it is not tidy, it cannot be kept clean.

16.4 Maintenance and Service Personnel

Through lack of training or supervision, people who enter a cleanroom to maintain or service machinery can be a considerable hazard. The maintenance technician, unless instructed otherwise, will apply the same techniques as they do outside the cleanroom. Service personnel from outside firms may be completely untrained in cleanroom contamination control techniques. The following is a list of procedures that should be considered for maintenance and service personnel:

- Maintenance and service technicians should only enter a cleanroom with permission.
- Maintenance and service technicians should be trained in cleanroom techniques, or closely supervised when they are within the cleanroom.
- Technicians must wear the same, or equally efficient, cleanroom clothing as cleanroom personnel, and use the same techniques to change into cleanroom clothing when entering and exiting cleanrooms. They should never enter the cleanrooms (especially at weekends, or when no one else is around) without changing into cleanroom clothing.
- Technicians should ensure they remove dirty boiler suits, etc. and wash their hands before changing into cleanroom clothing.
- Tools that are used routinely for maintaining the cleanroom should be cleaned (and sterilised, if required) and kept stored for sole used within the cleanroom. Tools should be made from materials that do not corrode. For example, stainless steel is much preferred to mild steel tools , which may rust.
- If a service engineer or contractor brings tools into the cleanroom (especially those from outside the cleanroom organisation), then they must be cleaned. A wipe-down with a cleanroom wiper moistened with isopropyl alcohol (often 70%, in water) is a suitable method. Only the tools or instruments needed within the room should be selected, decontaminated, and put into a cleanroom compatible bag or container. This has the advantage of leaving behind cases or briefcases, with their associated scraps of paper, fluff etc., which are potential sources of contamination; these should not be allowed into the room.
- Spare parts or items, like fluorescent light tubes, which have wrappings, should have the wrappings removed outside the manufacturing area and the parts wiped down. Information on this topic is given in Sections 18.3 and 18.4.

- Written methods should be kept for each activity, so that contamination control techniques can be incorporated within a specification. These should be adhered to.
- Any instructions or drawings on non-cleanroom paper must not be taken into the cleanroom. They can be photocopied onto cleanroom paper, or laminated within plastic sheets, or placed in sealed plastic bags.
- Particle generating operations such as drilling holes, or repairing ceilings and floors should be isolated from the rest of the area. A localised extract or vacuum can also be used to remove any dust generated.
- Technicians should not bring any materials into a cleanroom that are given on a list of 'contaminating material', similar to that in the list in Section 18.1 of this book.
- Technicians must tidy up when they are finished and ensure that the area is then 'cleanroom cleaned' by a person with suitable knowledge. Only cleaning agents, materials and equipment that has been approved for use in the cleanroom should be used.

Acknowledgement

I would like to thank Lynn Morrison for posing for the photographs contained within this chapter.

17

Entry and Exit of Personnel

People can disperse millions of particles and thousands of microbe-carrying particles from their skin and clothing. It is therefore necessary for personnel working in a cleanroom to change into clothing that minimises this dispersion.

Cleanroom clothing is made from fabrics that do not break up and lint; they therefore disperse the minimum of fibres and particles. Cleanroom clothing also acts as a filter against particles dispersed from the person's skin and their indoor, or factory, clothing.

The type of cleanroom clothing used varies according to the type of cleanroom. In cleanrooms where contamination control is very important, personnel wear clothing that completely envelops them and prevent their contamination being dispersed, i.e. a coverall, hood, facemask, knee-length boots and gloves. In cleanrooms where contamination is not as important, less enveloping clothing such as a smock, cap and shoe covers may be quite sufficient. Information about cleanroom clothing is given in Chapter 19.

Whatever the choice of clothing, garments will have to be donned prior to entering the cleanroom, and they should be put on in such a way that the outside of the clothing is not contaminated. This chapter describes typical methods.

Some types of cleanroom garments are worn once before being thrown away; others are sent for cleaning and processing after being used once. However, garments are normally used more than once. It may therefore be necessary to devise a storage method to ensure that a minimum of contamination is deposited onto them. Possible methods are discussed at the end of this chapter.

17.1 Prior to Arriving at the Cleanroom

Poor personal cleanliness is not acceptable in a cleanroom. However it is not clear how often personnel should bathe or shower, there being little in the way of scientific investigations into this topic. Clearly a shower would be necessary if someone has just had a haircut and is likely to shed hair clippings. It is known that washing can remove the natural skin oils and, in some individuals, the dispersion of skin and skin bacteria can increase. People with dry skin may wish to use a skin lotion to replace the lost skin oils.

Consideration should be given to what clothing is best worn below cleanroom garments. Clothing made from artificial fibres, such as polyester, are better than those made from wool and cotton, because synthetic fabrics disperse much fewer particles and fibres. Close-woven fabrics are also an advantage, as these are more effective in filtering and controlling the particles and microbe-carrying particles dispersed from the skin. This type of problem will be overcome if personnel are issued with factory undergarments. These should be made from a fabric that does not lint, and it should effectively filter particles dispersed from the person.

Personnel should consider whether applying cosmetics, hair spray, nail varnish, etc. at home is necessary, as these should be removed prior to entering the cleanroom. They should also consider what rings, watches and valuables they will bring to work, as they are likely to be removed and stored. These and other suggestions with regard to staff entering a cleanroom are discussed in Section 16.1.

17.2 Changing into Cleanroom Garments

The best method of changing into cleanroom garments is one that minimises contamination getting onto the outside of the garments. One such method is described below. Some of the suggested procedures may be unnecessary in poorer classes of cleanrooms, and further procedures can be introduced in cleanrooms that manufacture products very susceptible to contamination. It should also be noted that alternatives to the proposed method are successfully used in existing cleanrooms, and these are quite acceptable as long as they give a level of contamination control appropriate to the standard of the cleanroom.

The design of clothing change areas is discussed in Chapter 5 where it is explained that the change area is normally divided into zones. These may be rooms, or rooms divided by crossover benches. Change areas can vary in design, but it is common to find them divided into three zones:

(1) Pre-change zone
(2) Changing zone
(3) Cleanroom entrance zone.

Personnel move through the zones in the following manner.

17.2.1. Approaching the pre-change zone

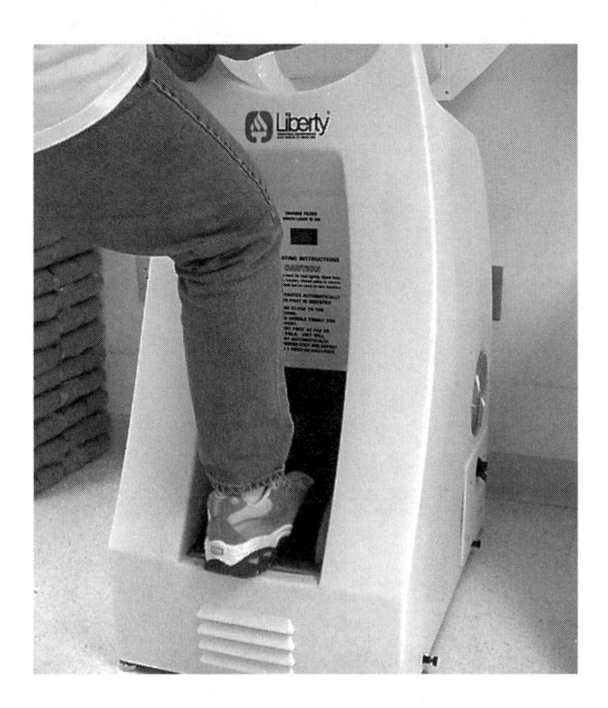

Figure 17.1 Cleanroom shoe cleaner

Before starting to change into cleanroom clothing, it is best that personnel blow their nose. It is impossible to do this correctly in a cleanroom, and if this is done it will save an unnecessary trip out of the cleanroom. They should also go to the toilet. If it is necessary to come out of the cleanroom to go to the toilet, it is likely to entail changing out and back into cleanroom clothing.

In cleanrooms where outdoor shoes are not removed, or effectively covered, shoe cleaners should be used. Cleanroom shoe cleaners are specially made to retain contamination dispersed from the shoe: use of one is illustrated in Figure 17.1.

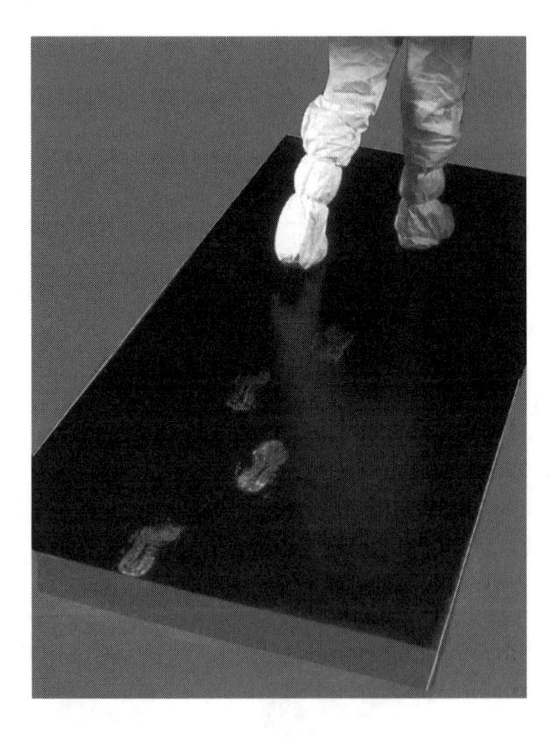

Figure 17.2 Dycem cleanroom mat

Sticky cleanroom mats or flooring are often used in the approach to the change room. These are specially manufactured for use in cleanrooms. There are two general types. One type is laminated from layers of thin adhesive plastic film and the other from a thick resilient adhesive plastic.

Both work by removing dirt from the soles of footwear as personnel walk over them (see Figure 17.2). After a while they become soiled. In the case of the plastic film version, the topmost layer is peeled off to expose a fresh layer. In the case of the resilient plastic type the surface is washed.

If a laminated mat is used, shoes should be applied to a mat three times to ensure the removal of practically all of the footwear contamination. If the resilient-type cleanroom flooring is used it can cover a floor surface area large enough to ensure that sufficient steps are placed on it to ensure effective dirt removal. This is a minimum of three per foot i.e. six in all.

17.2.2 Pre-change zone

Within the pre-change zone the following tasks may be carried out:

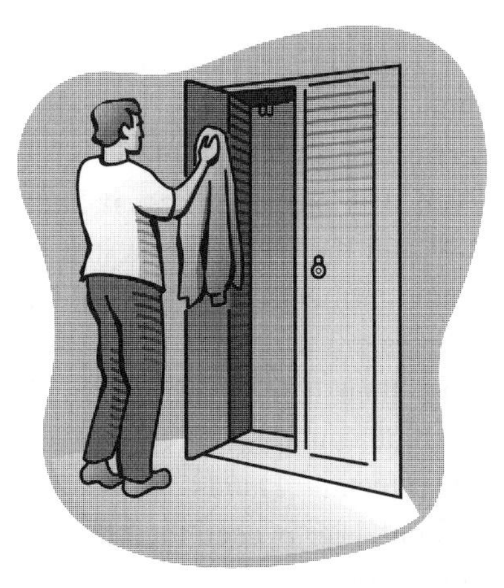

1. Personnel should remove sufficient street or factory clothes to feel comfortable in the cleanroom. If the company provides dedicated clothing to wear under the cleanroom garments, then all street clothing should be removed and replaced with factory garments.

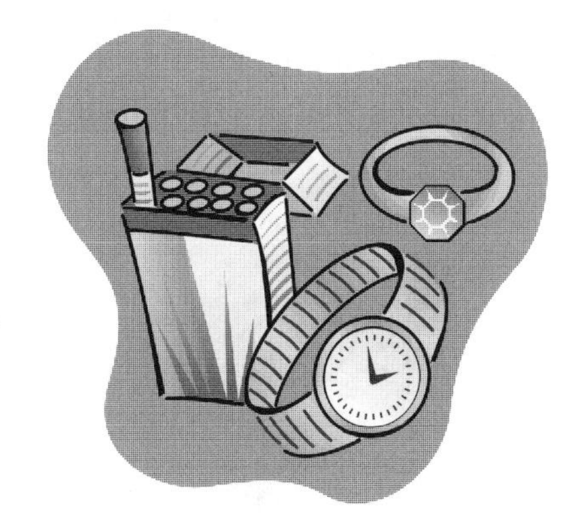

2. Watches and rings should be removed. They can harbour dirt, produce chemical and particle contamination, and are liable to tear gloves. Wedding rings that are smooth may be kept on if the ring (and under the ring) is kept clean. Rings that are not smooth can be taped over. Items such as cigarettes and lighters, wallets and other valuables should be securely stored.

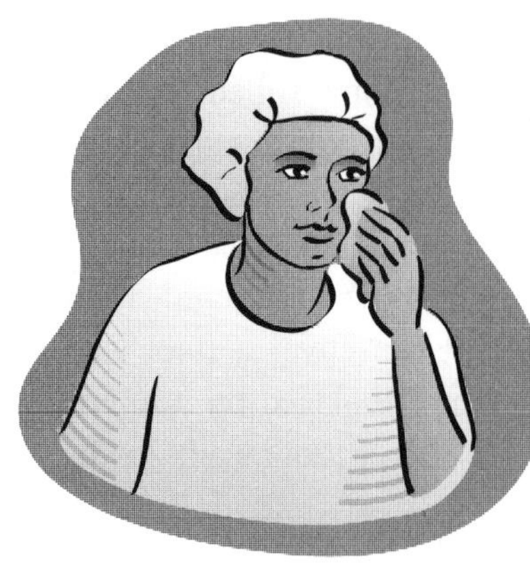

3. Remove cosmetics and, if required, apply a suitable skin moisturiser. The composition of any moisturiser should be considered to ensure that no chemicals used in the formulation cause contamination problems in the product being manufactured.
4. Don a disposable bouffant hat, or hairnet. This ensures that hair does not stick out from under the cleanroom hood.
5. Put on a beard cover, if appropriate.
6. Put on a pair of disposable footwear coverings, or change into dedicated cleanroom shoes.

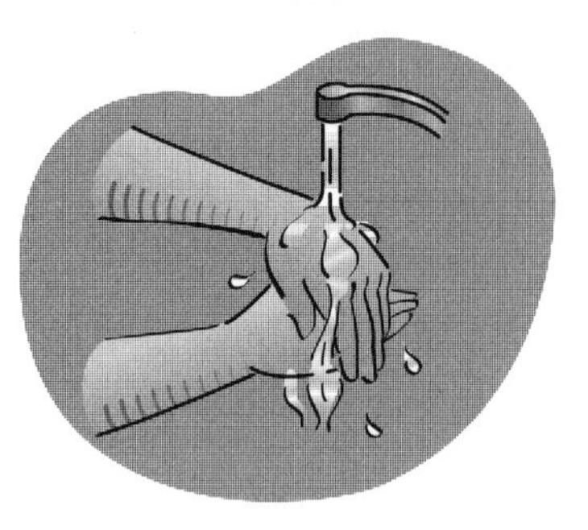

7. If a hand washing system is located in this area then wash the hands, dry them and, if necessary, apply a suitable hand lotion. However, it is probably best if hands are washed within the change area just before the clean garments are put on (see below). If gloves are used to put on cleanroom clothing, then hand washing can be done here. In bioclean areas, it will be necessary to wash the hands in a suitable skin disinfectant. Hands can be dried with a non-linting towel or a hand drier. If a hand drier is used then the best type is one that does not disturb the dirt on the floor.

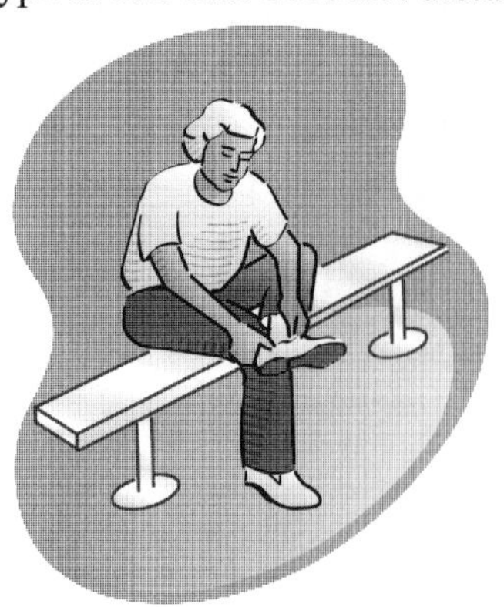

8. Cross over from the pre-entry area into the change zone. The demarcation between these two zones may be a door or a crossover bench, or both. A sit-on transfer bench may be built across the zones to ensure that personnel cannot walk round but must cross over it. If a bench is used footwear should be attended to as it is crossed. If a bench is not used, then a cleanroom mat or flooring should be used. Personnel

should stop at the mat and put their footwear three times to the mat to make certain that it is clean and the minimum of contamination is tracked into the next zone.

17.2.3. Changing zone

The garments used in the cleanroom are put on in this area. Several methods can be used but the following is suggested. This uses a method assumes that a facemask, hood, coverall and overboots are used, but it can be adapted for use with a cap, gown and overshoes. It requires that the garments are put on from the top down.

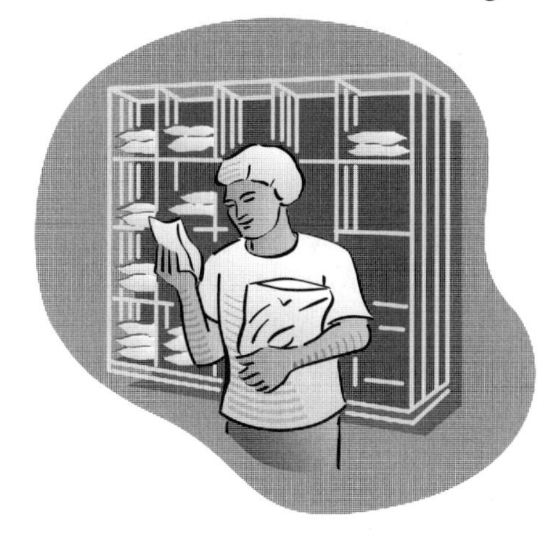

1. The garments to be worn are selected. If a fresh garment is used, then it should be checked for size and the packaging checked to ensure that it is free from tears and faulty heat seals. The packaging is then opened.
2. A facemask and hood (or cap) is put on. It appears to make little difference whether the mask is put under, or over, the hood. Choose which method is the most comfortable. If a hood is put on, the hair must be tucked in and the studs (snaps) or ties at the back of the hood adjusted for comfort.
3. If a hand washing system is installed in this area then the hands should now be washed (and disinfected if required). This is possibly

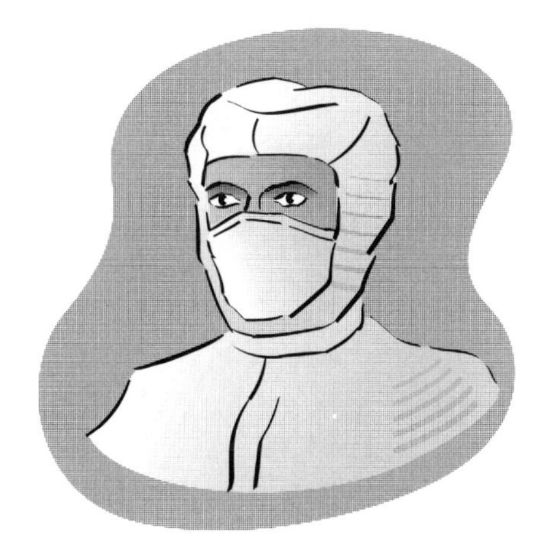

the best time for personnel to wash their hands as clean garments will now be handled and contaminated parts of the body, such as the hair and face, should not be touched again.

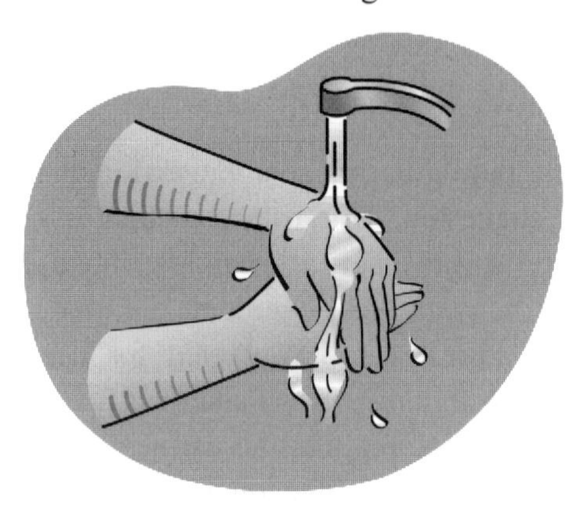

4. Temporary gloves known as 'donning gloves' are sometimes used to prevent the outside of the cleanroom garment being contaminated. Use of these gloves is confined to the higher quality of cleanroom. These should, if required, be put on.

5. The coverall (or gown) should be removed from its packaging and unfolded without touching the floor. It is sometimes possible to get the cleanroom laundry to fold the garment in a way that will minimise both the chance of the garment touching the floor and the outside surface being contaminated by the personnel's hands. If this is not done, then the following can be considered.

If a coverall is used, it should be removed from its packing and allowed to unfold without touching the floor. It should be unzipped and turned so that the zip is to the side away from the person.

There are now several methods of putting on the garment to ensure that it does not touch the floor. These are as follows:

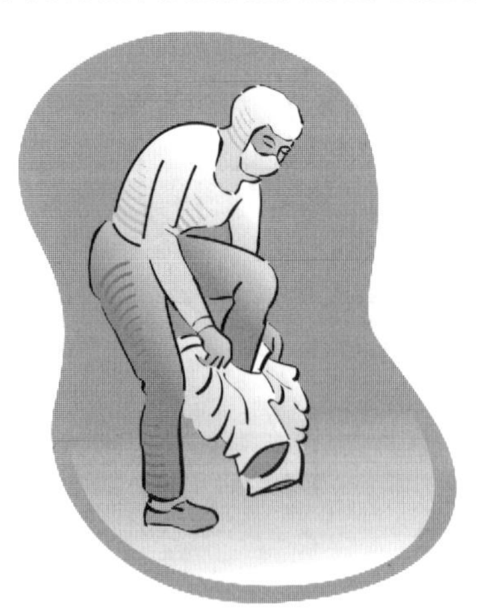

- The coverall can be gathered together at the 4 corners i.e. the two wrists and the two ankles. It should then be possible to put first one leg and then the other into the garment without the trouser legs touching the floor.
- The garment can be held in the inside at waist level, some of the material gathered up and one leg and then the other put in to the trouser legs. The top of the coverall can then be slipped over the shoulders, or,

- The left cuff and left zipper can be taken in the left hand and the right zipper and right cuff taken in the right hand. The coverall can then be gathered up at the waist and one leg placed into the garment, and then the other leg placed into the other garment leg. By releasing one cuff at a time, first one arm and then the other can be placed into the garment.

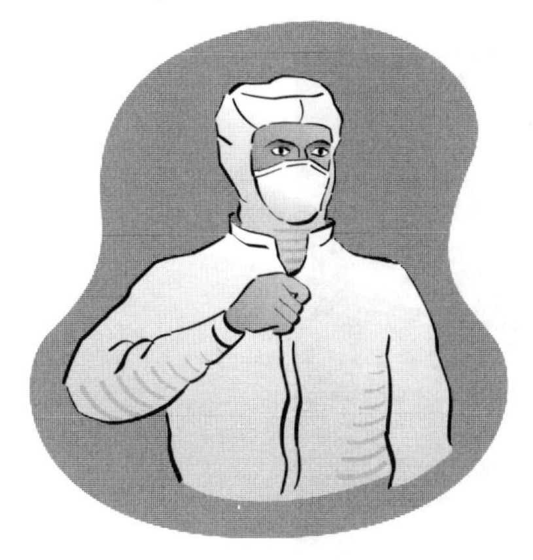

The last two methods will work better if the trouser legs are folded back on themselves so that they are shorter and less likely to touch the floor. The garment should then be zipped all the way up to the top, ensuring that all of the hood (if used) is tucked under the collar. A mirror is useful at this stage.

If the garment has press studs (snaps) at the ankles and wrists, then these should be snapped shut.

17.2.4 Cleanroom entrance zone

1. If a crossover bench is available, it should be crossed over now. This bench is used to demarcate the slightly soiled changing-zone from the cleaner entrance zone, and allows cleanroom footwear (overshoes or overboots) to be correctly put on.

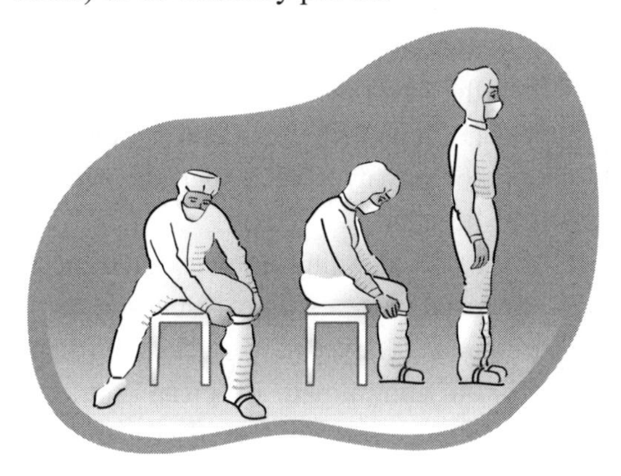

2. Personnel should sit on the bench. One leg should be raised, the cleanroom footwear put on, the leg transferred over the bench and placed on the floor of the entrance zone. Then the other leg should be raised, the cleanroom footwear put on and the leg taken over the bench. While still sitting on the bench, the legs of the cleanroom garment and the footwear

should be adjusted for comfort and security. Personnel should now stand up.

3. If required, protective goggles of the type shown in Figure 17.3 can be put on. These are used not only for safety reasons but to prevent eyelashes and eyebrow hair falling onto the product.

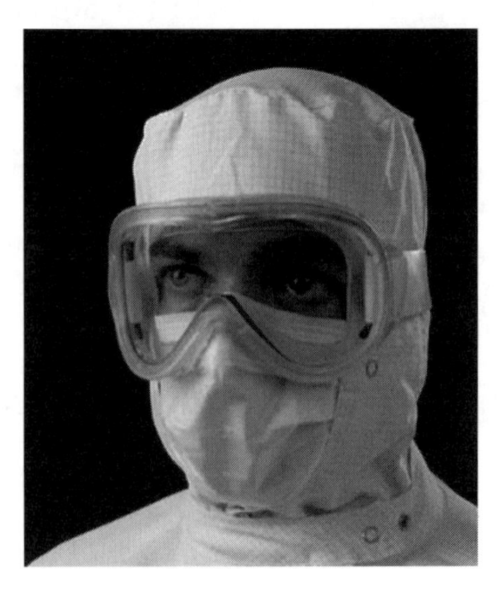

Figure 17.3 Protective goggles

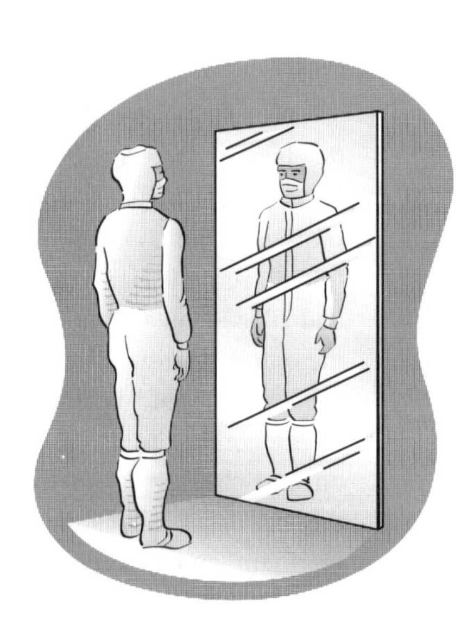

4. The garments should be checked in a full-length mirror to see that they are worn correctly. Check that the hood is tucked in and there are no gaps between it and the coverall (or gown). Check that no hair can be seen.

5. If donning gloves have been used they can be dispensed with now. They can, however, be kept on and a pair of clean working gloves put on top. Two pairs of gloves can be used as a precaution

against punctures, although sensitivity of touch is lost.

6. If deemed necessary, the hands can again be washed. Gloves can also be washed. In a biocleanroom it is beneficial to decontaminate the hands by applying an alcohol solution containing a skin disinfectant. Apart from being more efficient, the use of an alcohol solution overcomes the problem of having a washhand basin in the room, with its attendant risk of microbial growth.

7. Low particle (and if required, sterile) working gloves should now be put on, without the outside of them becoming contaminated. In some cleanrooms this task is left until the personnel is within the production cleanroom. If they are latex gloves, which are wrapped in pairs with the cuffs rolled back (in the style used by surgeons), then the gloves can be put on without being contaminated. In this case, the first glove is taken out of the exposed package by gripping the fold of the rolled-over cuff with the one hand and inserting the other hand into it. Two fingers of the gloved hand are then passed under the rolled-over cuff of the second glove and it is lifted from the package. The hand is then put into the second glove, the fingers being slotted into the correct fingers of the glove, and the cuff lifted over the cuff of the cleanroom garment. It is now possible to pull back the cuff of the first glove, making sure that it is completely over the garment's cuff.

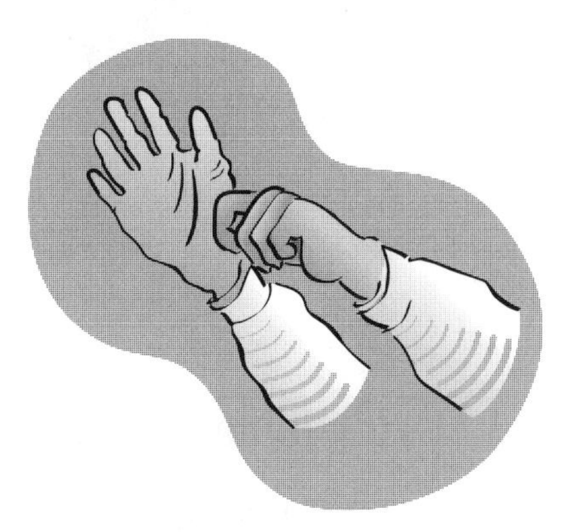

8. Most cleanroom gloves are not packed in a way that will allow gloves to be put on without contaminating the glove surface. These gloves must be gripped at the edge of the cuff and put on in a similar way to that described above. Gloves packed in pairs will be contaminated less than those packed in 50s or 100s, as it is difficult to remove a glove from a large pack without contaminating those that are left. If considered necessary, the gloves can now be washed or disinfected.

9. Personnel may now proceed into the cleanroom. This may be over a cleanroom mat.

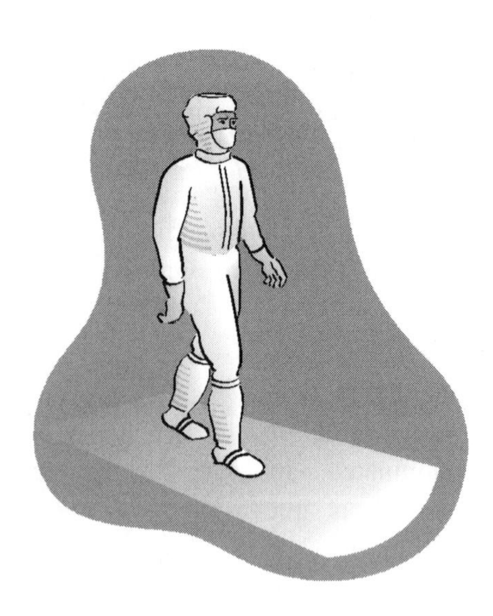

17.3 Exit Changing Procedures

When leaving a cleanroom, personnel will either (i) discard all their garments and on re-entry use a new set of garments (this is normally only employed in an aseptic pharmaceutical cleanroom), or (ii) discard their disposable items, such as masks and gloves, but reuse their coverall, smock, etc. on re-entry.

If a complete change of clothing is required on re-entry, then the disposable items such as bouffant hats, gloves, facemask and disposable overshoes are placed in a container for disposal. If the remainder of the garments are not disposable then they should be placed in a separate container for dispatch to the cleanroom laundry for processing.

If the garments are to be used again on re-entry, they should be removed so that the outside of the garment is contaminated as little as possible. The cleanroom footwear should be removed, one at a time, at a cross-over bench, as each leg is taken over the bench. The coverall should then be unzipped and removed using the hands within the garment to remove it over the shoulder and down to the waist. In a sitting position, one leg is now removed the garment. The empty arm and leg of the garment should be held so that they do not touch the floor. The other leg can now be removed. The facemask and hood can now be removed.

Garments to be used again on re-entry should be stored to prevent contamination. This can be done in several ways, as follows:

- Each item of clothing can be rolled up. In the case of cleanroom footwear this should be done so that the dirty soles are to the outside. The footwear can now be placed in separate pigeon holes and the hood and coverall (or cap and gown) in another. If thought necessary, the items of clothing can be placed into bags before being put into the pigeon holes.
- The hood (or cap) can be attached to the outside of the coverall (or gown) by means of a snap (stud) and hung up, preferably in a cabinet. The cleanroom footwear can be placed at the bottom of the cabinet. It is best that their garments should not touch the wall, or each other. In higher grade cleanrooms, clothing is often hung up in unidirectional flow cabinets (see Figure 5.7 in Chapter 5), specifically designed to ensure that garments are not contaminated.
- Garment bags can be used. These will have separate pockets for the various clothing items and should be regularly laundered.

Acknowledgements

The cartoons used to illustrate this chapter are used the kind permission of CleanRooms Magazine, a PennWell Publication. Figure 17.1 is reproduced by permission of Roger Diener of Analog Devices Inc. Figure 17.2 is reproduced by permission of Dycem Ltd. Figure 17.3 is reproduced by Metron Technology.

18

Materials, Equipment and Machinery

18.1 Choice of Materials

Materials used in cleanrooms must be selected with care to ensure that they do not contribute to the contamination in the room. Typical of materials used in a cleanroom are:

- Materials used in the manufacturing. In a pharmaceutical manufacturing area it might be containers and ingredients. In the microelectronics industry it might be silicon wafers and process chemicals;
- Packaging for the product. This could be, for example, glass or plastic bottles, plastic bags and pre-formed boxes;
- Process machinery and equipment;
- Tools used for the maintenance, calibration or repair of equipment and machinery;
- Clothing for personnel, such as suits, gloves and masks;
- Materials for cleaning, such as wipers and mops;
- Disposable items such as writing materials, labels and swabs.

Depending on the products made in the cleanroom, contamination on materials can be:

- particles
- micro-organisms
- chemicals

- electrostatic charge
- molecular outgassing.

In almost all cleanrooms, particles and fibres will be a problem. Materials that break up easily or disperse particles when used in the manufacturing process should therefore be avoided. Materials that come into cleanrooms with particles or fibres on their surface should also be avoided. In bioclean rooms of the type used in the healthcare and food industries, micro-organisms are contaminants. In the semiconductor industry chemicals, both on the surface and outgassed, may deposit onto the surface of a semiconductor, and are a problem. Materials that are unable to continually conduct away any electrostatic charge may cause difficulties in some cleanrooms if the charge builds up and discharges to an electrically sensitive product. A static charge may also attract particles to the material, and these can cause contamination problems.

Materials used in cleanrooms for manufacturing should be chosen not only because they are suitable for manufacturing, but because of their non-contaminating properties. Materials and items that are required for production, but are clearly contamination sources, should be used only if essential, and only if these contamination control problems have been recognised and alternative steps considered and rejected.

Depending on the susceptibility of the product to contamination, some, or all, of the following list will be prohibited because of contamination problems:

- abrasives or powders;
- aerosol-producing cans or bottles;
- items made from wood, rubber, paper, leather, wool, cotton and other naturally occurring materials that break up easily;
- items made from mild steel, or other materials that rust, corrode or oxidise;
- items that cause problems when machined or processed, e.g. they may smoke or break up;
- paper not manufactured for use in cleanrooms. If ordinary paper must be used then it should be sealed in plastic envelopes or laminated between plastic films;

- pencils and erasers;
- writing implements such as fibre-tipped pens that could scratch paper, or whose ink contains contaminating chemicals;
- paper correcting fluid;
- personal items listed in Section 16.2 should not be brought in by cleanroom personnel;
- disposable items such as swabs, tapes and labels that are not cleanroom compatible.

Items used for cleaning the cleanroom such as wipers, mops and cleaning solutions should be selected from a range that have been specially manufactured for use in cleanrooms. This is discussed in Section 20.3. Similarly, maintenance and test tools, such as spanners and screwdrivers, should be selected to minimise contamination, and should be kept clean.

18.2 Items Supplied from Outside Manufacturing Sources

Items can arrive in a cleanroom badly contaminated if they come from a supplier who is not knowledgeable or concerned about cleanroom requirements. This can, in some instances, be the single most important cause of contamination of products, and steps may have to be devised to overcome the problem.

Items supplied for use in a cleanroom should ideally be manufactured in a cleanroom of the same standard as the cleanroom they are used. They should also be produced using similar cleanroom contamination control techniques. If items cannot be delivered with a suitable level of cleanliness, then they will then have to be cleaned within the cleanroom; this is unlikely to be as effective. The number of firms who produce components in cleanrooms is growing, but many have manufacturing conditions that are less than ideal. It may be possible to persuade your supplier to adopt suitable contamination control measures. If your company, or the total cleanroom industry, has sufficient buying power, the manufacturing company may wish to safeguard their market by producing products of the appropriate degree of cleanliness.

A visit to the premises of your supplier to audit their facilities is essential. The manufacturer may not be acquainted with cleanroom technology, and some simple suggestions and changes to their manufacturing process may produce useful dividends. Even if the manufacturer has no cleanroom, a higher level of housekeeping, the use of cleanroom gloves, wipers and non-linting clothing may make a considerable difference to the quality of the product. Attention should also be paid to storage and packaging. If the product can be taken from the production machine and immediately wrapped in suitable clean packaging, the effect of the poor surrounding conditions is minimised: this may be sufficient for your purposes.

18.3 Wrapping Materials

Wrapping of cleanroom items should not only prevent damage during transportation, but minimise contamination. An example will illustrate this. If a component is placed into a cardboard box and delivered to a cleanroom then its outside will be contaminated with wood fibres. Even if the component is put into a clean plastic bag before being placed in a cardboard box, the outside of the plastic bag will be contaminated with wood fibres; it will then be very difficult to open the bag without getting fibres onto the component. This problem can be overcome if the packaging is made from clean materials and multi-layered.

Plastic materials are most common materials used for packaging; they are often used either as a film or as pre-formed packaging. Plastic packaging is usually lower in particles, fibres and chemical contamination than many other materials. However, this does not mean that plastic materials are free from contamination. The amount of contamination will depend on the plastic used, and the manner it is made and packaged; its suitability should be checked.

Some plastics can produce an electrostatic charge that will harm the product. Static-dissipative plastic is available, and this has the additional advantage of being less likely to attract particles to it, and may therefore be cleaner. Some plastic packaging, such as that made from PVC, may not be acceptable if outgassing is considered a problem.

The number of layers of packaging should be considered. If an item used in a cleanroom is wrapped in multiple layers, then it is possible to remove a layer at a time as the materials progress into the cleanroom. This will ensure that items will arrive into the cleanroom cleaner. Vacuuming and damp wiping of the packaging is a useful method, especially in the initial entry stages. However, as the supplies pass into the cleanroom and the packaging gets progressively cleaner, it may become less necessary to clean the outside of the packaging. The following practical example will illustrate one possible approach.

Small items for use in a cleanroom are manufactured and packed singly in a pre-formed plastic pack. Groups of ten of these single packs are put into a plastic box with a lid and this is vacuum packed in plastic film. These are then put into a large plastic bag that is placed into a cardboard box for delivery. When the cardboard boxes are delivered to the factory where they are to be used, they are stored in some unclassified storage area for eventual use. When required, the cardboard box is taken to an area outside the materials-transfer airlock and the large plastic bag taken out. The bag can then be vacuumed with a brush attachment. The bag is opened and the vacuum-packed boxes removed and loaded onto a trolley. The trolley is taken into the materials-transfer airlock where the vacuum-packed wrapping is wiped with a damp cleanroom wiper. The wrapping is then cut open and the plastic boxes deposited onto a clean pass-over bench in the airlock; the wrapping should be cut open in such a way as to prevent contamination on the outside of the wrapping getting onto the clean inner items. If the top of a package is cut in a 'X' or an 'I' shape and the end corners cut down to the bottom of the package it should be possible to strip back the packaging without causing contamination. This is illustrated in Figure 18.1.

The plastic boxes on the pass-over bench are then picked up by cleanroom personnel and taken into the cleanroom. These will then be stored in the cleanroom. When a component in the pre-formed packaging is required the plastic box is opened, the item removed, and the lid shut.

The correct method of packaging of items varies a great deal depending on the items being packaged, their use, and the design of the materials airlock. It will therefore be necessary for the cleanroom management to specify suitable packaging materials and devise a protocol for cleaning and

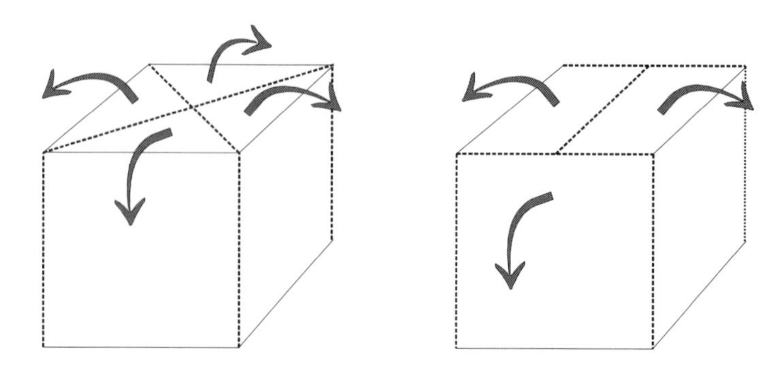

Figure 18.1 Cutting methods

removing the layers of packaging as the required item progresses into the cleanroom

18.4 Transfer of Items and Small Pieces of Equipment through an Airlock

Items used in manufacturing should be transferred into the cleanroom so that the minimum allowable contamination enters the cleanroom.

An airlock prevents air exchange into the cleanroom. A description of airlocks and their function is discussed in Section 5.2.1. When both sets of airlock doors are shut, the supply air dilutes the contamination that enters either through the door from the outside corridor, or is dispersed by the people using it.

It is common to find that the outer and inner doors of the materials transfer airlock are interlocked. This is done to ensure that one door cannot be opened until the other one is closed, and this prevents contamination in the outside uncontrolled area being directly transferred into the cleanroom. Cleanroom mats are used at the entry to an airlock, and sometimes into the cleanroom; these prevent the transfer of contamination on the soles of shoes' or the wheels of trolleys (carts).

An airlock is also used to prevent the entry of contamination on the surface of the materials, and their packing. Given below is a description of two possible methods that can be used to transfer materials through an airlock.

Depending on the type of materials being transferred and the security of the transfer, either a 'no-bench' or a 'bench' method is used. These are discussed below.

18.4.1 Transfer area with a bench

A secure method of transferring supplies into a cleanroom is to use an airlock divided into two zones by a bench. This is not a suitable method for transferring heavy materials and equipment, and an alternative method is discussed in the next section. If a bench is used the following method may be employed.

The door from the uncontrolled area is opened and the person enters. The person may walk over a cleanroom mat or flooring to minimise the transfer of outside floor contamination. The pass-over bench is cleaned and, if necessary, disinfected (Figure 18.2).

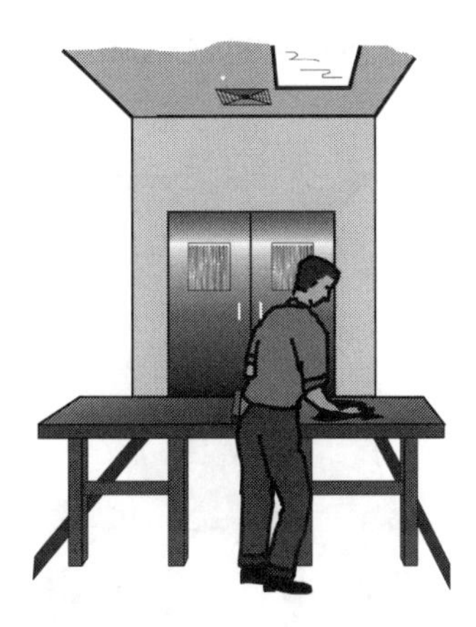

Figure 18.2 The bench is cleaned

The wrapped items are now brought into the air lock. No packaging material that will cause gross contamination, such as cardboard, should be brought into the airlock. The package should be placed on the 'wrapped receiving' or 'dirtier' part of the pass-over bench (Figure 18.3).

The wrapping is then cleaned and removed (Figure 18.4); this method depends on the standard of cleanroom being accessed, and is discussed in Section 18.2.

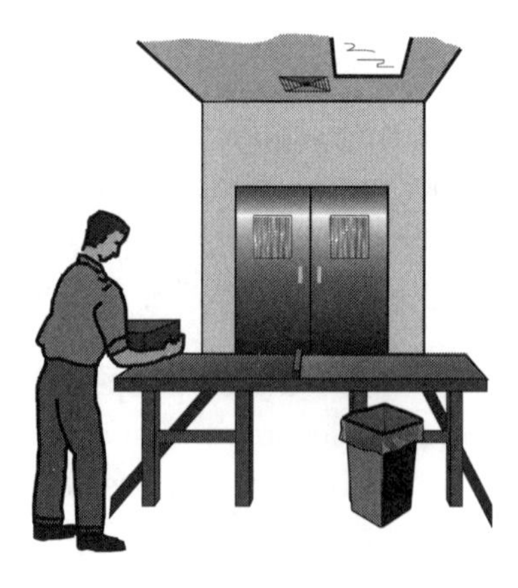

Figure 18.3 Wrapped items placed on 'wrapped receiving' side of bench

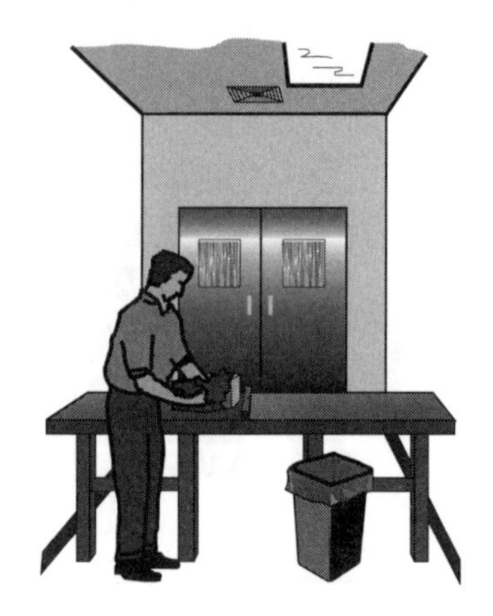

Figure 18.4 Wrapping removed

The outer packaging is now removed and deposited into a suitable container. The item is then be placed on the 'wrapping removed' or 'clean' part of the bench (Figure 18.5).

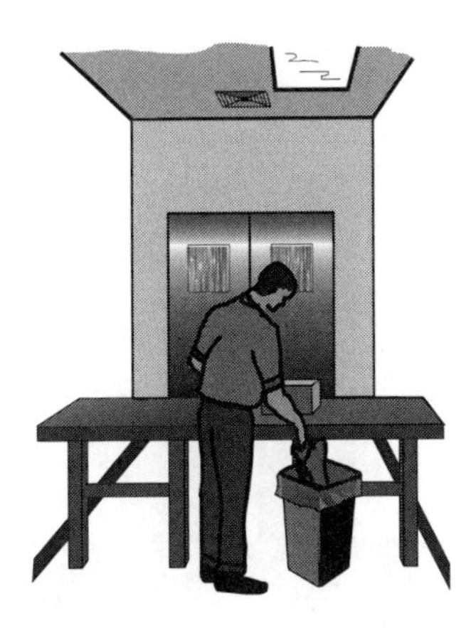

Figure 18.5 Unwrapped item place on clean side of bench

The person who has brought in the materials from the outside area will then leave. The airlock may be left for a few minutes to allow the airborne contamination to come down to a concentration that does not significantly affect the cleanroom when the door into the cleanroom is opened. A timer on the door interlocks or light may assist this. Cleanroom personnel now enter the cleanroom and pick up items that have been left (Figure 18.6).

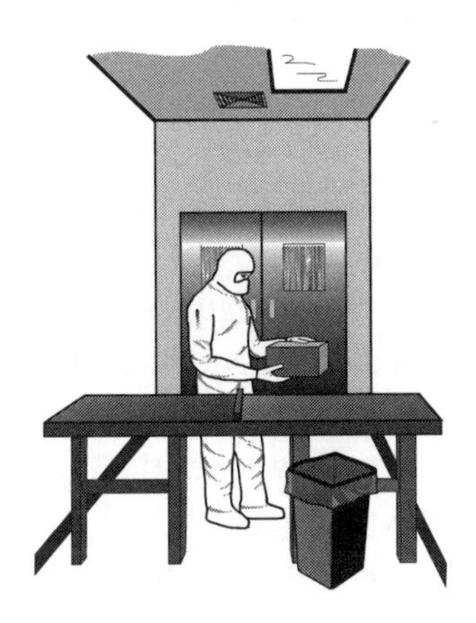

Figure 18.6 Cleanroom personnel pick up the material

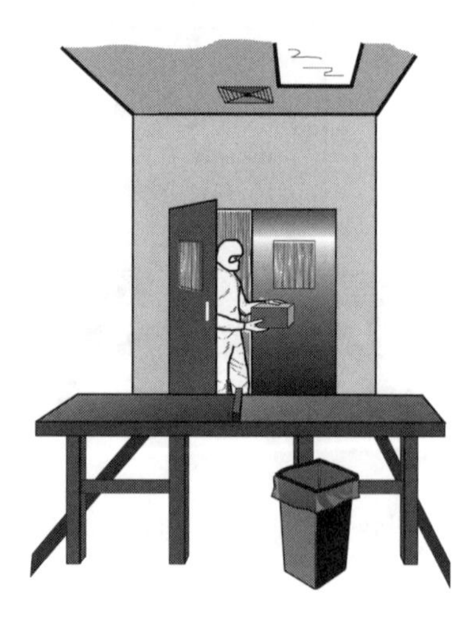

Figure 18.7 Material taken into cleanroom

Cleanroom personnel then pass back through the inner door and into the cleanroom (Figure 18.7).

18.4.2 Transfer area without a bench

An airlock without a bench is often used if it is necessary to pass large heavy pieces of equipment or machinery in and out of the room. It can also be used as a less secure alternative to an airlock with a bench. Such a type of airlock is illustrated in Figure 18.8.

Using the methods discussed in the previous sections of this chapter, a clean trolley, or cart, is loaded with materials for use in the cleanroom. It is pushed from the outside uncontrolled area into the transfer airlock and left. Personnel from the cleanroom then enter the transfer area to get the supplies. If the supplies are heavy and cannot be lifted, the trolley will have to enter the cleanroom; it will have to be cleaned in the airlock before this occurs. If the supplies are not heavy, then they can be transferred to a cleanroom-designated trolley that has been brought from the cleanroom for this purpose.

Using a method similar to that discussed in previous sections of this chapter, the item's packaging is cleaned, or removed, or both. The cleanroom trolley (cart), is then taken into the cleanroom and the doors closed. Depending on whether the trolley is required for removing out-going goods, or to bring in more supplies the 'outside' trolley can be removed, or left.

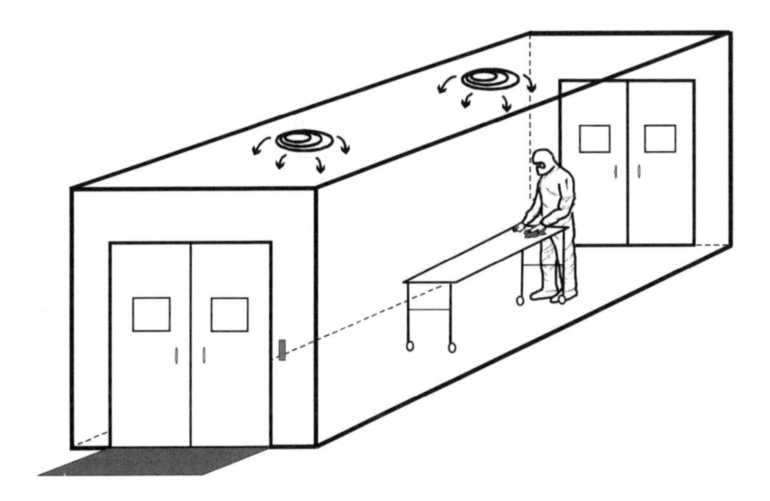

Figure 18.8 Material-transfer area suitable for a trolley or bulky machinery

It may be considered necessary to use a cleanroom mat or flooring to remove the contamination from the wheels of the trolley (cart), as it is pushed into the cleanroom.

18.5 Entry of Machinery

Machines, and other heavy and large bulky items of equipment, are occasionally taken in or out of a cleanroom. The method to do this should have been established when the cleanroom was designed. Unfortunately, this is not always done.

The best solution to the movement of bulky items is to design the materials airlock to be large enough to allow the entry and exit of every piece of machine to be brought in or out of the room. As has been discussed in the previous section, the materials airlock may be divided into two parts by the bench. If it is anticipated that the chance is small of a large machine being brought in or out of the cleanroom, then the bench system can still be used. However, the bench should not cause an obstacle by being (a) designed with the floor covering passing up and over it, (b) permanently attached to the floor, or (c) with a lip on the floor.

Another design solution for getting machinery in and out of a cleanroom is to provide a set of double doors in the cleanroom wall that are large enough for the machinery or plant items to pass through. These are likely to give direct access to the outside corridor, and must therefore be locked, except when needed for the entry of machinery. Some types of modular wall panels can be removed and replaced without disruption, and this is an alternative to doors. Both these methods are not as good as an airlock, as it is not possible to ensure that the machinery is clean when it enters the cleanroom, or that outside contaminated air will not get into the cleanroom. It will therefore be necessary when the machinery has been placed in the cleanroom to clean the machinery, clean the cleanroom and then carry out tests to ensure that the disruption has not compromised the cleanroom's cleanliness.

It is quite common in established cleanrooms to find that the materials airlock is too small for machinery, there is no doorway in the wall, and that wall panels cannot be easily removed. Sometimes it is possible to get the machinery through the changing rooms, but if the materials airlock is too small, it is likely that the changing area is as well. In this situation, there are two possible solutions:

1. Cut a panel in the wall of the production room so that the machinery can pass through from the outside corridor. This hole in the wall can then be reinstated, preferably with double doors for future use. After the machinery has been commissioned, the cleanroom can then be cleaned, tested and production restarted. This method cannot be used if production must continue in the cleanroom. It is also particularly ineffective if it has been necessary to effect an entry through materials that disperse copious amounts of contamination, such as plaster panels or bricks and mortar.
2. A temporary airlock can be constructed on the inside surface of the wall of the cleanroom. For better security, an airlock should be built on both

sides. The wall can then be penetrated and a doorway built in the wall. If these airlocks are now effectively cleaned and cleanroom mats used to minimise foot-borne transfer, they can be use to test and clean the machine before it passes into the cleanroom. If this method is expertly done, it is possible to continue production within the cleanroom during the modifications.

The equipment used to lift the heavy machinery and similar items into a cleanroom is unlikely to be suitable for cleanroom use. It can be cleaned, but this is unlikely to be sufficient. It may therefore be necessary to cover the lifting equipment with clean plastic film that is taped in place.

18.6 Transfer of Materials through Hatches and Sterilisers

Items for use in a cleanroom can be transferred into cleanrooms by methods other than a materials transfer airlock. A popular means of transferring small items in or out of a cleanroom is by the use of a transfer hatch. The actual size of the hatch will depend on the size of the materials being transferred, but the transfer hatch shown in Figure 18.9 has doors approximately 90cm by 90 cm and a depth of about 40 cm.

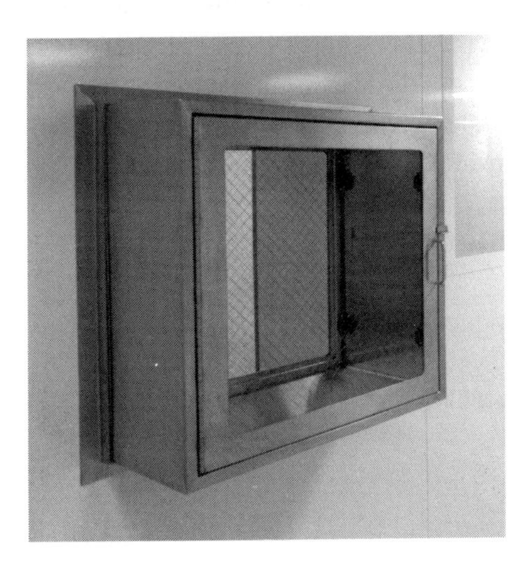

Figure 18.9 Pass-through hatch

The transfer hatch works in a similar way to a materials airlock. If an item is passed into a cleanroom, the following method may be used:

- The person outside the cleanroom opens the transfer hatch door and cleans the hatch.
- A layer of packaging is taken off and the item placed into the pass-through hatch.
- The door is shut.
- The person on the other side of the hatch opens the inner door and removes the item. These items may be cleaned, or another layer of packaging removed if higher contamination control is required.

It is common to find that the transfer hatch has an electrical or physical type of interlock that prevents the two doors being open at the same time, and thus preventing an undesirable exchange of air into the cleanroom. Hatches can also be constructed at floor level. This allows heavier items to be more easily transferred through the hatch.

Sterilisers, such as autoclaves and hot air ovens, are used to transfer materials in and out of biocleanrooms. To do this efficiently, double-door sterilisers, are used. The door outside the cleanroom is opened and the non-sterile material is loaded into the steriliser. The steriliser then proceeds through its sterilising cycle. After it is complete the steriliser door into the cleanroom is opened and the sterilised materials removed. It is also possible to use sterilising tunnels, where containers are sterilised as they pass from the outside to the inside of the cleanroom.

Acknowledgement

Figure 18.9 is reproduced by permission of Thermal Transfer.

19

Cleanroom Clothing

Large amounts of contamination are dispersed from the people in clean-rooms. Special clothing is therefore worn in all cleanrooms to control the particle and microbiological dispersion from people and hence the con-tamination within cleanrooms.

The use of clothing to reduce the dispersion of contamination origi-nated in hospitals. At the end of the 19th century it was realised that sur-geons who inspected patient's infected wounds in hospital wards trans-ferred bacteria-containing pus and blood onto their clothing. When they moved to the operating room they infected wounds.

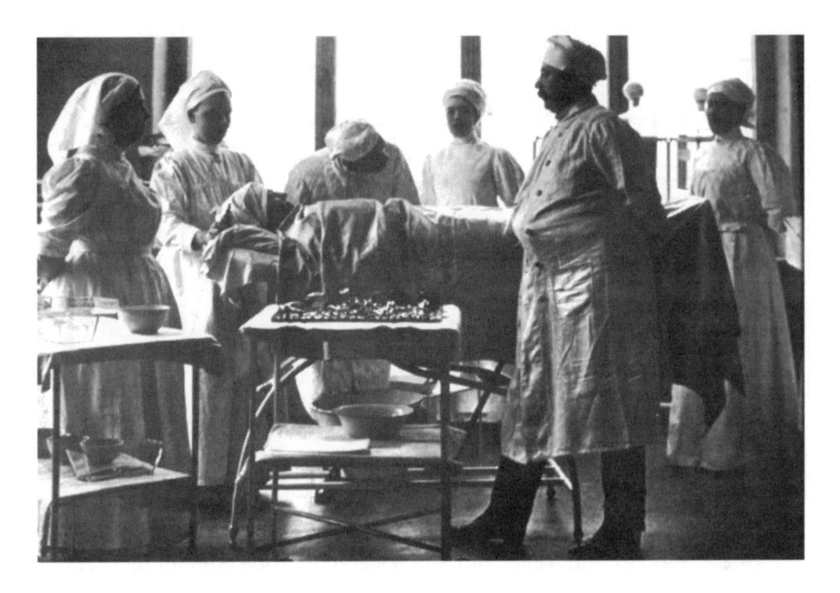

Figure 19.1 Old operating room clothing.

To protect the patient's wound during surgery, sterile gowns were used. Figure 19.1 shows an old operating room where the surgeon in the forefront of the picture can be seen wearing a sterile gown over his normal clothes.

How airborne contamination is dispersed, and the role of cleanroom clothing in reducing this, can be conveniently considered in two parts, i.e. inert particles and microbe-carrying particles.

19.1 Sources and Routes of Inert Particle Dispersion

The airborne dispersion rate from people varies from person to person, the greater their activity the more particles they disperse. Dispersion is dependent on the clothing worn, but can be in the range of 10^6 to 10^7 per minute for particles ≥ 0.5 µm, i.e. up to 10^{10} per day.

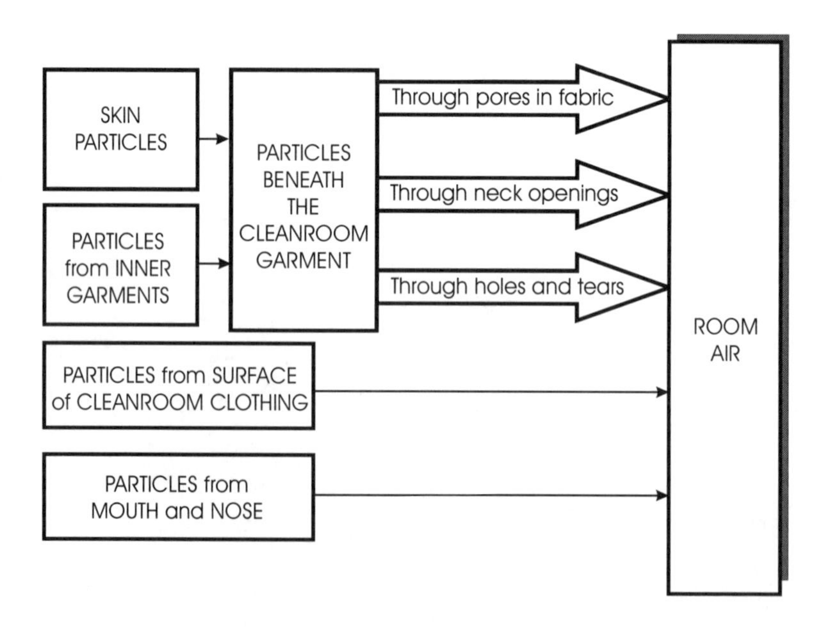

Figure 19.2 Sources and routes of particles and microbe containing particles from people

People may disperse particles from:

- skin
- clothing they wear under cleanroom garments
- cleanroom clothing
- mouth and nose.

The routes of dispersion of particles are through the following parts of cleanroom clothing:

- fabric
- poor closures at the neck, ankles and wrists
- holes and tears.

These routes and sources shown in Figure 19.2, are those that occur when coveralls are worn. However, when coats or smocks are worn, there is no barrier between a person's legs and the bottom edge of the coat, and contaminated is freely dispersed from underneath.

19.1.1 Sources of particles and mechanisms of release

The sources of particles are listed in the previous section and shown in Figure 19.2. These are now discussed in more detail in relation to their importance and the mechanisms of releasing particles.

19.1.1.1 Skin

People shed approximately 10^9 skin cells per day. Skin cells are approximately 33µm × 44 µm and found in the cleanroom either as whole cells or fragments. Figure 19.3 shows a photograph of the surface of the skin taken by means of an electron microscope. The lines shown in the photograph delineating the individual skin cells and beads of sweat on the surface. The amount of sweat shown is equivalent to that generated by one hour of exercise.

Skin cells may be released onto clothing and laundered away; others are washed away in the bathtub or shower. However, a large number are

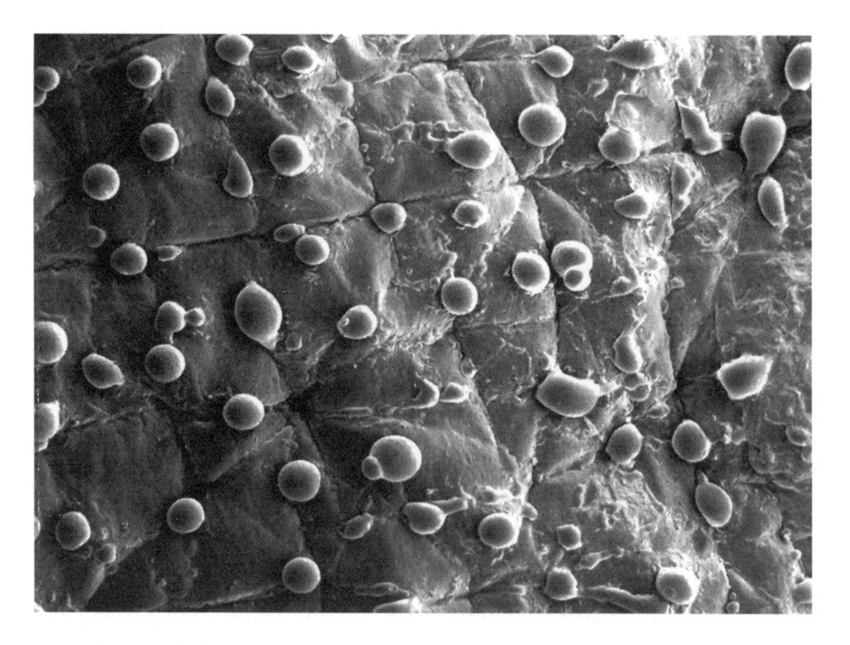

Figure 19.3 Skin surface showing skin cells and beads of sweat

dispersed into the air. These skin particles are a major source of airborne contamination.

19.1.1.2 Clothing under cleanroom clothing

What people wear under their cleanroom garments has a large effect on their inert particle dispersion rate. If their inner clothing is made from natural fabrics, such as a cotton shirt, cotton jeans and woollen jersey, they disperse large quantities of particles. The reason for this is that these natural materials have fibres that are both short and break up easily.

Figure 19.4 shows a photograph of the structure of cotton, and it is not difficult to envisage fragments of the fibres breaking off. These fragments then combine with the dispersed skin particles and pass through the outer cleanroom garment. However, if the inner clothing is made from synthetic fabric, the particle challenge from the inner garments can be reduced by 90% or more. It can be reduced even more if the inner garment has a good filtration efficiency against the skin particles.

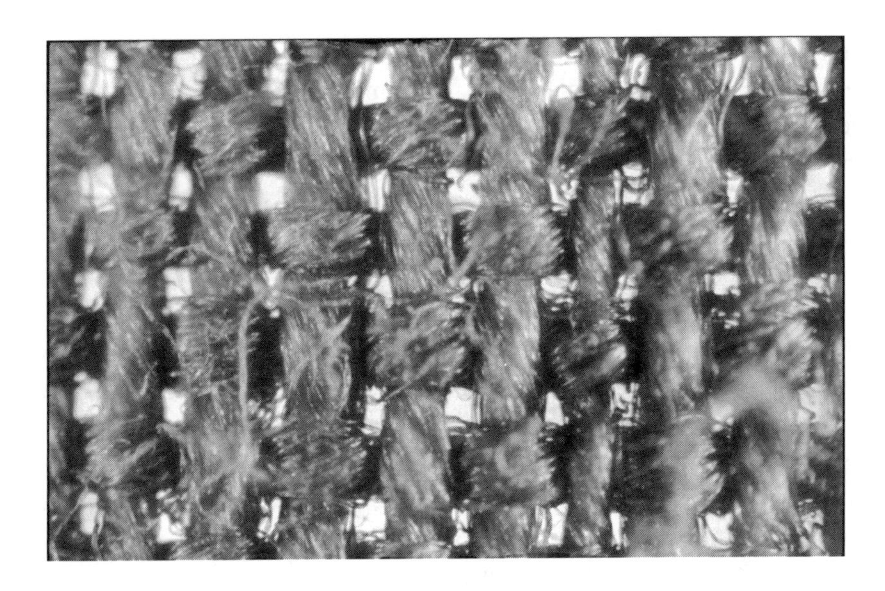

Figure 19.4 Cotton fabric photographed through a microscope. Magnification about 100 times

19.1.1.3 Cleanroom clothing

The cleanroom industry has placed considerable emphasis on minimising the particles dispersed from cleanroom clothing, i.e. on non-linting properties of the fabric and the cleanliness of the clothing. As will be discovered from further reading of this chapter, this is overemphasised. Although natural fabrics, such as cotton, give off an unacceptable number of particles, these are never (and must never be) used in cleanrooms.

Cleanroom clothing is made from fabrics manufactured from synthetic plastic materials, such as polyester or nylon. These fabrics are unlikely to break up when used in cleanroom clothing, and have been shown to contribute about only 5% of the total number of particles dispersed by a person; the majority of particles come from a person's skin or inner clothing.

Figure 19.5 shows a photograph of the structure of a synthetic cleanroom fabric. It can be seen that the fabric is woven from threads made from continuous synthetic monofilaments, and this ensures that few particles are dispersed from the fabric.

19.1.1.2 The mouth and nose

People will disperse particles from their mouth or nose. When people sneeze, cough or talk, they emit particles. Snorting through the nose also disperses particles. These mechanisms, and the means of preventing them, are discussed in Chapter 20.

19.1.2 Routes of transfer of particles

Although a fabric of the type shown in Figure 19.5 sheds few particles by breaking up, they do little to prevent particles passing through them. The pores at the intersection of the threads of this fabric are between 80μm and 100μm, this being caused by the monofilaments having a large diameter and the fabric not being woven tightly. The particles generated from the skin and the inner clothing therefore pass through easily. This is therefore not a desirable cleanroom clothing fabric. A cleanroom fabric should be manufactured so that it can prevent particles passing through. This is discussed later in Section 19.3.

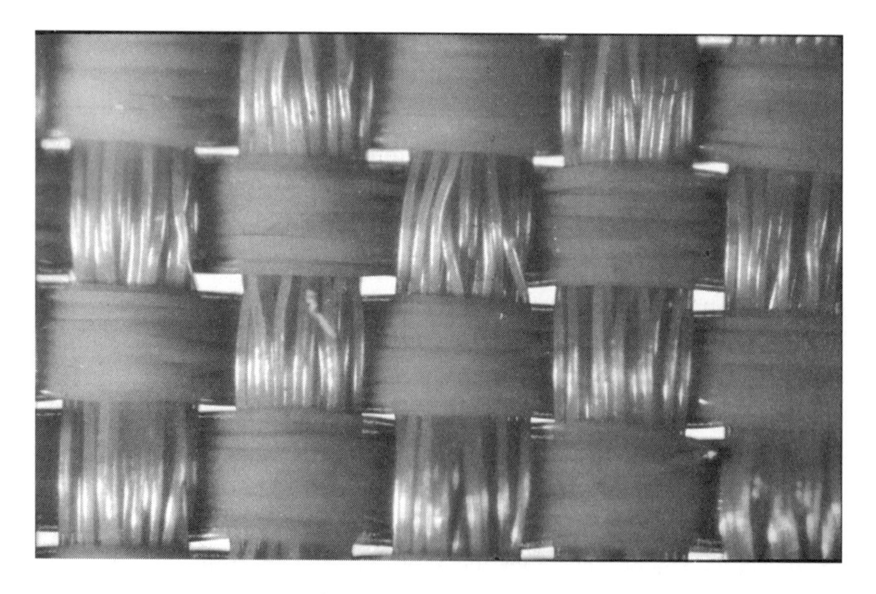

Figure 19.5 A poor cleanroom fabric with large pores (about 80μm to 100 μm equivalent diameter) between the threads

As personnel move, a pressure builds up under the cleanroom clothing. The pressure is greater as the air impermeability of the fabric increases. The particles under the cleanroom clothing may then be pumped out of closures at the neck, ankles, wrists and zips. Secure closures can prevent this, and although they should be tight, they should not be uncomfortable.

If a garment has tears or holes, particles can easily pass through. If a garment such as a smock is worn, it will not fully envelop a person and particles flow out from under it and into the cleanroom.

19.2 Routes and Sources of Microbial Dispersion

The sources and routes of microbe-containing particles from people are the same as with inert particles and shown in Figure 19.2. However, the relative importance of the microbial sources is different.

19.2.1 Sources of micro-organisms

People are normally the only source of micro-organisms in a cleanroom. Almost all of the airborne micro-organisms found in the cleanroom air come from people's skin, although some come from the mouth and nose. Information on dispersion from the mouth and nose is discussed in Chapter 20.

People shed one outermost layer of epithelial cells every 24 hours. A small but significant proportion of these is dispersed into the cleanroom air with micro-organisms on them. Micro-organisms grow and divide on the skin, and can be found as either a small microcolony, or individual cells.

Figure 19.6 shows a microcolony on the skin with about 30 bacteria in it. The majority of skin cells dispersed into the environment do not have micro-organisms on them. On average, about one in ten of the skin cells dispersed have micro-organisms on them; they are likely to have an average of about four microbes on each. The type of micro-organisms on airborne skin cells is almost always bacteria, this being a reflection of the type of microbes found on the skin.

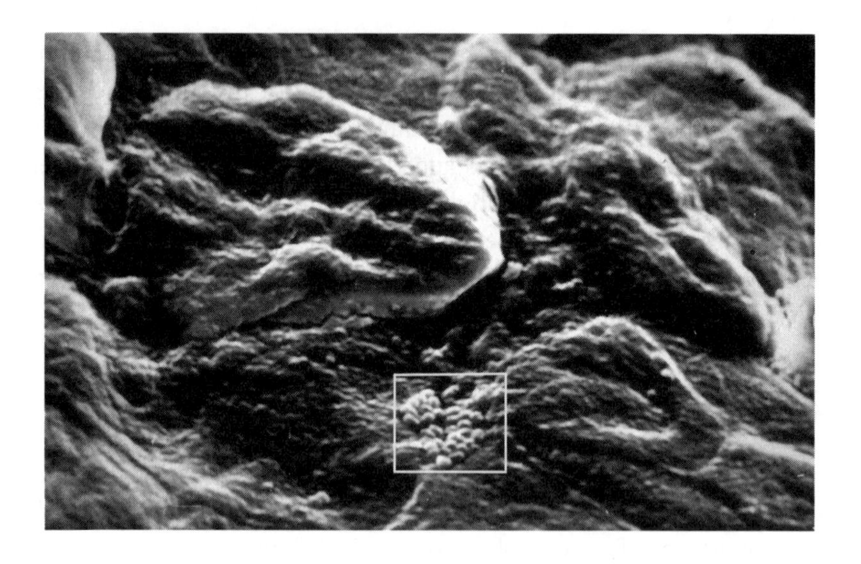

Figure 19.6 Microcolony of bacteria on surface of skin

Most microbe-carrying particles in the air of a cleanroom come from the skin. Large numbers of inert particles come from the person's inner clothing and small numbers from the break up of cleanroom clothing. These two sources are not primary sources of microbe-carrying particles.

19.2.2 Routes of microbial dispersion

The routes of transfer through cleanroom clothing are the same as with inert particles and shown in Figure 19.2. These are:

- the pores in the fabric
- poor closures at the neck, sleeves and ankles
- damage to the fabric, i.e. tears and holes.

Microbe-carrying particles are also expelled from the mouth. When a person is breathing, microbial dispersion is too low to be measured but speaking, coughing and sneezing produce significant numbers. This is discussed in the next chapter.

People disperse large numbers of microbe-carrying cells. When males wear ordinary indoor clothing, an airborne dispersion rate of 1000 microbe-carrying particles per minute is not unusual, the average rate being closer to 200 per minute. Females will generally disperse less.

Closely-woven fabrics are more effective in reducing microbial than inert particle dispersion. The reason for this is that the average size of microbe-carrying skin cells is much larger than the inert particles found in the air. Microbe-carrying particles in cleanroom air have a size spectrum from less than 1 μm to over 100 μm, with an average equivalent diameter of between about 10 μm and 20 μm. They are therefore small enough for many of them to pass through the pores in cleanroom fabrics

19.3 Types of Cleanroom Clothing

19.3.1 Clothing designs

The most effective type of cleanroom clothing is that which completely envelopes a person. It should also be made from a fabric that has effective filtration properties and have secure closures at the wrist, neck and ankle. However, this type of clothing can often be the least comfortable and most expensive.

The choice of clothing will depend on what is being produced in the cleanroom. A poorer standard of cleanroom may use a cap, zip-up coat (smock) and shoe covers (Figure 19.7).

In a higher standard of cleanroom a one-piece zip-up coverall, knee-high overboots and a hood that tucks under the neck of the garment will be typical (see Figure 19.8). A spectrum of design exists around these two general types of garments.

Some of the best cleanroom clothing can be 10 times more costly than the most basic. However, it can be cost effective to buy good cleanroom clothing. It is not unusual for a firm to pay several million dollars, or pounds sterling, for a new cleanroom that is used by less than ten people. The firm’s buyer may then purchase the cleanroom clothing. They may be ignorant of the function of clothing and refuse to spend a little extra money to buy clothing that will achieve a drop in bacterial or particle contamination similar to that achieved by the new cleanroom.

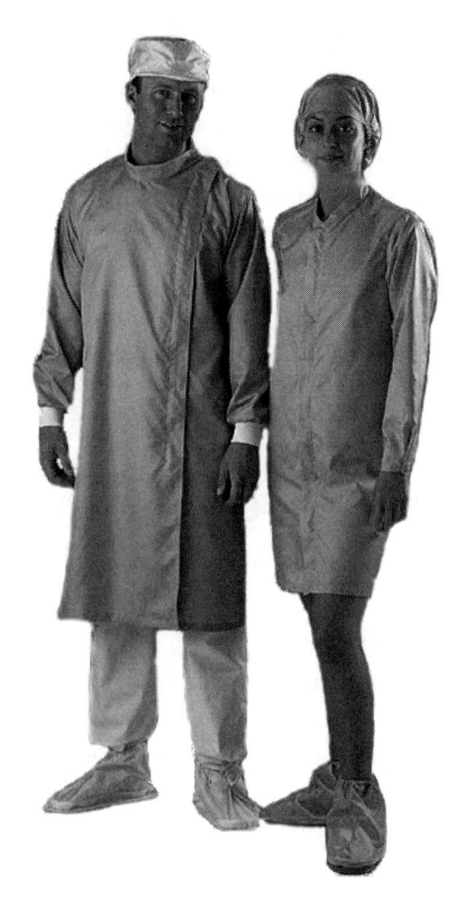

Figure 19.7 Cleanroom garments suitable for a lower standard of cleanroom

19.3.2 Cleanroom fabrics

The type of fabric is an important consideration when choosing a cleanroom garment. Cleanroom fabrics should be resistant to break-up (linting). A more important property is their ability to filter the contamination generated from the skin and clothes worn under the cleanroom clothing. The fabric's effectiveness can be assessed by measurement of the air permeability, particle retention, and pore-size. These tests are discussed in Section 19.6.

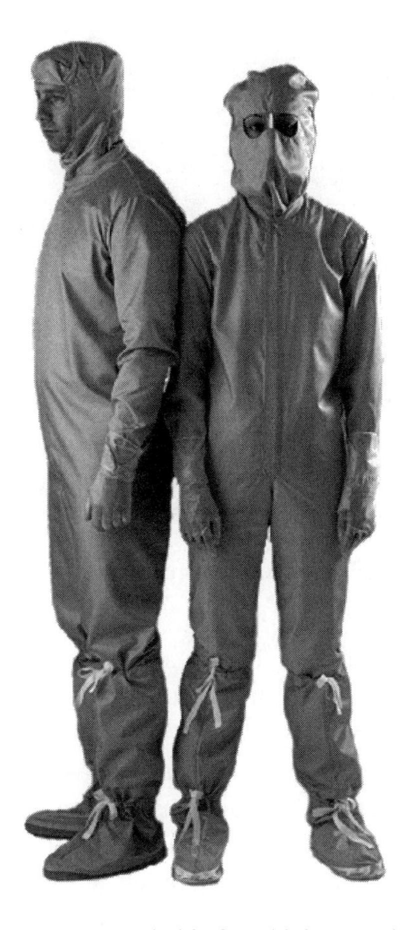

Figure 19.8 Cleanroom garments suitable for a higher standard of cleanroom

The most popular type of clothing is made from woven synthetic fabrics, the most common being polyester. This type of clothing is worn, processed in a cleanroom laundry and worn again. Figure 19.9 shows a cleanroom fabric that is made from finer monofilaments of polyester and is more tightly woven than the poor fabric shown in Figure 19.5; it is therefore a better particle filter. This type of fabric is similar to that often used in cleanrooms. However, more tightly-woven fabrics made from smaller diameter microfibres are also available. These work even better as long as the closures at the neck, ankles and wrists are able to prevent the extra pressure generated by the lower air permeability of these fabrics.

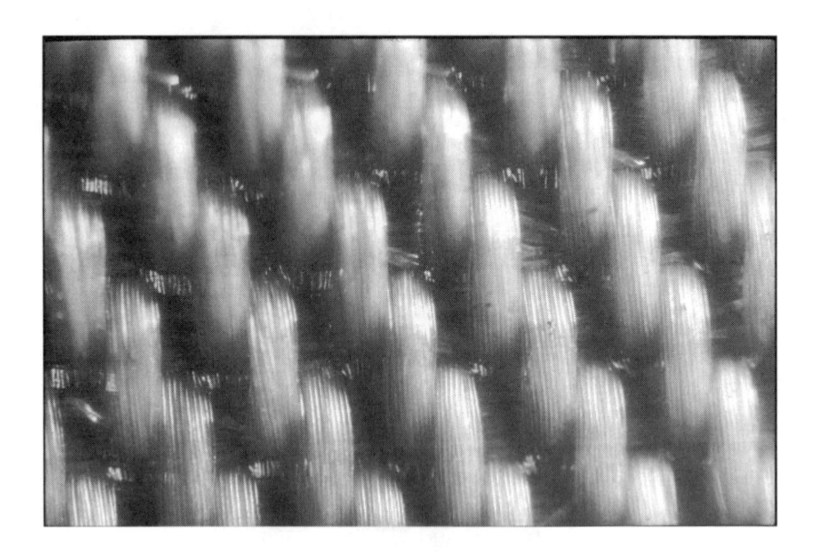

Figure 19.9 Typical construction of a cleanroom fabric

Non-woven fabrics, such as Tyvek, are used as single, or limited reuse, garments. They are popular for visitors and are used by builders when constructing the room. They are also popular in pharmaceutical manufacturing facilities in the USA. Other non-woven fabrics are successfully used in the manufacture of cleanroom garments. Membrane barrier fabrics, such as GoreTex, which use a breathable membrane sandwiched onto, or between, synthetic woven fabrics, are very efficient; they are expensive, and hence are used in the higher standard rooms.

The movement of a person generates an air pressure behind the garment fabric; the tighter the construction the higher the pressure. This will result in unfiltered air being pumped out of the closures of the clothing. Closures at the neck, cuffs and bottom of trousers must therefore be secure.

The number of holes and tears in garments must be kept to a minimum. If this is not done, contamination from the inner garments and skin will flow through unhindered. Garments should therefore be inspected at the laundry and before being put on. Any garments with holes or tears should not be used in a cleanroom. Care must also be taken to minimise holes in the garment by means of good construction.

19.3.3 Garment construction

To ensure good construction of cleanroom garments, the following methods should be used:

- To prevent the raw edges of the fabric fraying, the edges should be either covered, interlocked, heat seared or laser cut.
- To minimise contamination, the edges of the fabric should be encapsulated in seams. These seams should also minimise the escape of particles caused by needle punctures.
- To minimise contamination, the sewing threads should be made of synthetic continuous filament.
- To minimise shedding, the zippers, fasteners and shoe soles should not chip, break up or corrode. They should be able to stand up to multiple laundering and, where necessary, sterilisation.
- To prevent dirt collecting, there should be no pockets, pleats, darts or hook-and-pile fasteners (Velcro).
- To minimise contamination, elasticised or knitted cuffs should not collect or shed particles.

19.3.4 Choice of garments

The type of garments used in cleanrooms can vary. Information on the type of clothing that should be worn in different types of cleanrooms is given in the IEST Recommended Practice RP-CC-003.2. The information given in the Recommended Practice is summarised in Tables 19.1 and 19.2. Table 19.1 gives suggestions for different classes of cleanroom and Table 19.2 provides suggestions for aseptic cleanrooms.

Table 19.1 Garment systems for different classes of cleanrooms according to IEST-RP-CC-003.2

Apparel Type	ISO 7 & 8 (100K and 10K)	ISO 6 (1000)	ISO 5 (100)	ISO 4 & 3 (10 and 1)
Frock	R	AS	AS(NR*)	NR
2 piece suit	AS	AS	AS	AS
Coverall	AS	R	R	R
Shoe cover	R	AS	AS(NR*)	NR
Boot	AS	R	R	R
Special footwear	AS	AS	AS	AS
Hair Cover (bouffant)	R	R	R	R
Hood	AS	AS	R	R
Facial cover	AS	AS	R	R
Powered headgear	AS	AS	AS	AS
Woven gloves	AS	AS	AS	NR
Barrier gloves	AS	AS	AS	R
Inner suit	AS	AS	AS	R

R = recommended NR = not recommended
AS = application specific (NR*) = not recommended in nonunidirectional flow

Table 19.2 Garment systems for aseptic cleanrooms (IEST RP CC-003.2)

Apparel Type	ISO Class 7 (Class 10 000	ISO Class 6 and 5 (Class 1000 and 100)	ISO Class 4 and 3 (Class 10 and 1)
Frock	NR	NR	NR
2 piece suit	NR	NR	NR
Coverall	R	R	R
Shoe cover	NR	NR	NR
Boot	R	R	R
Special footwear	AS	AS	AS
Hair cover (bouffant)	R	R	R
Hood	AS	R	R

Facial cover	R**	R**	R**
Powered headgear	AS	AS	AS
Woven gloves	NR	NR	NR
Barrier gloves	R	R	R
Inner suit	AS	AS	R

R = recommended NR = not recommended
AS = application specific R** = surgical mask recommended

Information on clothing for pharmaceutical cleanrooms is also given in the European Union Guide to Good Manufacturing Practice (1997 edition). The type of clothing expected in the various grades of pharmaceutical cleanrooms is as follows:

> '*Grade D* [approximately equivalent to ISO Class 8 (Class 100 000)]:
> *Hair and, where relevant, beard should be covered. A general protective suit and appropriate shoes or overshoes should be worn.*
> *Grade C* [approximately equivalent to ISO Class 7 (Class 10 000)]:
> *Hair and, where relevant, beard and moustache should be covered. A single or two-piece trouser suit, gathered at the wrists and with high neck and appropriate shoes or overshoes should be worn. They should shed virtually no fibres or particulate matter.*
> *Grade A/B* [approximately equivalent to ISO Class 5 (Class 100)]:
> *Headgear should totally enclose hair and, where relevant, beard and moustache; it should be tucked into the neck of the suit; a face mask should be worn to prevent the shedding of droplets. Appropriate sterilised, non-powdered rubber or plastic gloves and sterilised or disinfected footwear should be worn. Trouser-legs should be tucked inside the footwear and garment sleeves into the gloves. The protective clothing should shed virtually no fibres or particulate matter and retain particles shed by the body'.*

19.3.5 Comfort

Cleanroom clothing can sometimes be hot and uncomfortable, and an effort should be made to maximise comfort. Clothing should therefore be provided in a selection of sizes. If the clothing is reusable it is quite common to have personnel measured and issued with their own clothing. The design of cleanroom garments should also provide closures at the neck, ankles and wrist that are a tight, yet comfortable.

Shoe coverings can cause problems. Simple, thin-plastic shoe-coverings can tear, fall off and stick to cleanroom flooring. If more substantial shoe coverings are selected, the sole should not mark flooring, or slip on wet floors. It is also important to find a good system of tying to ensure that they stay in place.

The thermal comfort of cleanroom garments can be assessed by, comfort indexes, such as water vapour permeability and Clo values. However, although these give an indication of comfort, it is best to get your personnel to try clothing out in your cleanroom. Inevitably, personnel will prefer garments that give the minimum of protection, as they are usually the most comfortable. It will be up to management to ensure that contamination control properties are pre-eminent, but a certain amount of trade-off may be necessary.

19.4 Processing of Cleanroom Garments and Change Frequency

19.4.1 Processing

Cleanroom clothing becomes contaminated during use and has to be replaced by fresh items. If disposable clothing is used it is simply thrown away, although some types can be processed a few times. If it is to be re-used, then it is usually cleaned in a cleanroom laundry. Other processes, such as antistatic treatment and disinfection or sterilisation, can also carried out by a cleanroom laundry.

Cleanroom laundries are built solely for processing cleanroom garments. A typical cleanroom laundry will have a design similar to that shown in Figure 19.10. There will be a 'soil area' where the garments are received and sorted out to minimise cross-contamination. Shoe covers will be separated. Some cleanroom managers are concerned to ensure that chemicals, or other toxic contaminants, are not transferred to or from their garments.

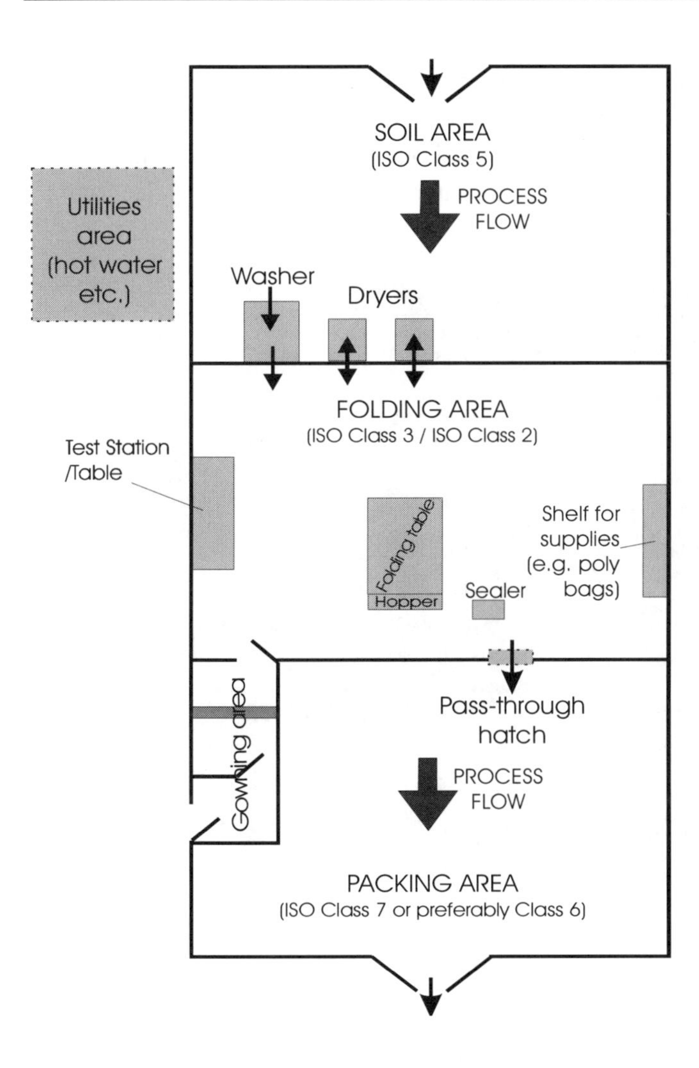

Figure 19.10 Diagram of a cleanroom laundry

The garments will then be put into a pass-through washer so dirty clothing can be fed into one side of the washer and clean garments emerge into the folding area. The washer will be fed with water that has been processed to purify it. Dry cleaning machines are also used. When the garments come out of the washing machine they will come into the folding area where the operators work in cleanroom garments. The cleanroom clothing is then loaded into a tumbler dryer that is supplied with filtered air. When dry, the cleanroom garments are inspected for holes or tears, folded and placed in clean bags. These are sealed and passed out of the folding area through a hatch into the packaging area for dispatch. A photograph of a cleanroom laundry in operation is shown in Figure 19.11.

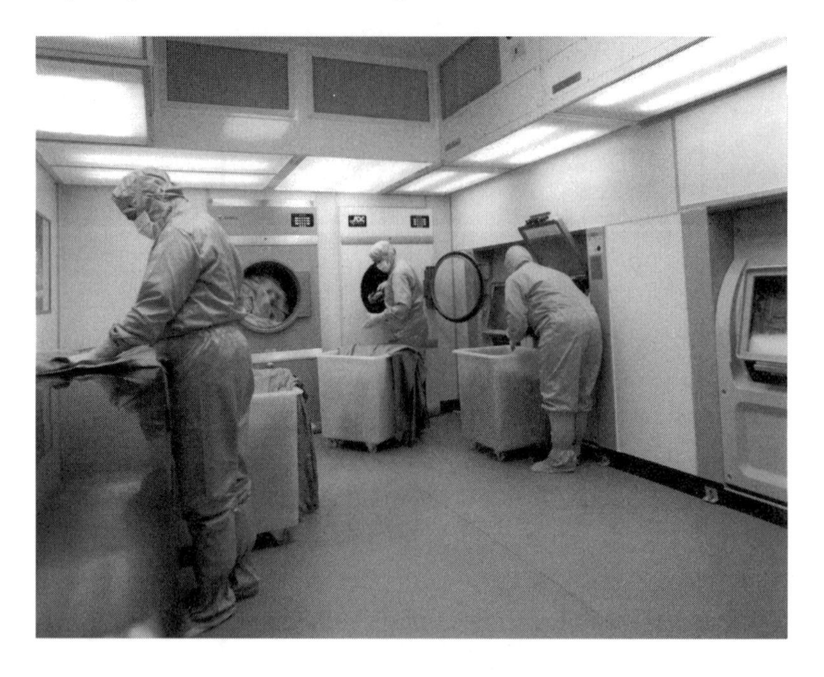

Figure 19.11 Cleanroom laundry showing the washers, tumble dryers and table for folding

If clothing is to be free of micro-organisms then the garments must be sterilised or disinfected. Sterilisation, i.e. the killing of all micro-organisms, can carried out by heat, gas or radiation methods. None of these methods is completely satisfactory. Autoclaving can cause substantial creasing and slow deterioration of the fabric. Gases such as ethylene oxide are gentler on the fabric, but their toxicity means that there can be problems with gas in the clothing and clothing must be left to off-gas.

Gamma radiation is a popular method, although this can cause discolouration of clothing and, in time, a breakdown of the materials. Another approach is to use disinfectants in the wash. This method should not damage the fabric and is more economical. However, it is possible that some micro-organisms may be left on the garment, and hence this method may not be acceptable.

The effectiveness of the cleaning process is normally checked by counting the number of particles on the surface on the processed garments. Samples are usually tested in the folding area (at the test station shown in Figure 19.10). Methods used are described in the IEST RP-CC-003, and are based on either the American Society for Testing of Materials (ASTM) F61 standard, or the tumbling drum test

19.4.2 Frequency of change

The frequency of the change of cleanroom clothing varies. One might expect that the more sensitive the process is to contamination, the more frequent the changing will be. However, this is not necessarily so. In the semiconductor industry where the cleanrooms are of the highest specification, clothing may be changed once or twice a week, with no apparent adverse effect in the airborne quality of the room. On the other hand fresh garments are put on every time personnel move into an aseptic pharmaceutical production area. Guidance as to the frequency of the change of garments in a typical cleanroom is given in the IEST RP-CC-003 and shown in Table 19.3.

Table 19.3 Recommended frequency of change of garment according to the IEST RP-CC-003

Class of Room	ISO 7 and 8 (Class 10 00 and 100 000)	ISO 6 (Class 1000)	ISO 5 (Class 100)	ISO 4 (Class 10)	ISO 3 (Class 1)
Frequency	2 per week	2 to 3 per week	daily	per entry to 2 per day	on each entry

19.5 The Effect of Laundering and Wear

In terms of particle removal efficiency, a garment is usually at its best when new. As it gets older the fabric will open up and allow more particles to be pumped through. The reason for this is that most cleanroom fabrics are calandered at manufacture by passing them through high-pressure rollers to squeeze the fabric and reduce the pore size. Fabrics that are more heavily calendered are more likely to relax through washing and use, and open up.

I have investigated the pore size and particle penetration of two garments when they were new and after being washed 40 times. One garment was made from a heavily calandered fabric, and its pore size increased from 17.2 μm to 25.5 μm, but the other identically woven fabric, which was less heavily calandered, only increased from 21.7 μm to 24.6 μm. A similar change in particle penetration was also observed. Clothing from one cleanroom user that was said to have been washed 'hundreds of times' had a pore diameter that increased from 18 μm, when new, to 29 μm. It is clear that the contamination control properties of garments can deteriorate with use and that some fabrics will be worse than others.

There is also a problem with holes and tears in the garments caused by accidents or wear. Personnel should check garments before they put them on; they should also be checked at the cleanroom laundry.

19.6 Testing of Cleanroom Clothing

Laboratory testing can assess the contamination properties of different types of clothing. The first type of testing is that of the *fabric*; these tests will ascertain its likely filtration properties. The second type of test is concerned with the performance of the *whole clothing system*; this is usually carried out in a body box. Further information on methods for testing clothing is given in the IEST RP-CC-003.

19.6.1 Fabric tests

My studies of the contamination control properties of cleanroom fabrics showed a wide variation in their properties. The equivalent pore diameter of varied from 17 µm to 129 µm, the air permeability from 0.02 to 25 $ml/s/cm^2$, the efficiency of removal of particles ≥ 0.5 µm from 5% to 99.99%, and particles ≥ 5.0 µm from <1% to 99.99%. This wide variation in the contamination control properties showed that care should be taken in choosing fabrics.

These laboratory tests identify fabrics that are likely to perform well when made into clothing. However to compare complete garments, a method that comes close to the real situation in a cleanroom is the body box test.

19.6.2 Dispersal of airborne bacteria and particles

The body box, which I first designed in 1968, is shown in Figure 19.12. Through a HEPA filter in the top of the box, bacteria and particle-free air is supplied. A volunteer enters the box wearing the clothing to be studied. After the contamination in the box has been blown out, the volunteer starts to exercise to the beat of a metronome. The number of particles and bacteria dispersed per minute are then counted. The usefulness of the body box is illustrated by some results.

19.6.2.1 Effect of the garment design on dispersion

Garments should be designed to envelop personnel and prevent the dispersion of contamination. The average number of the bacteria dispersed per minute from a male volunteer in a body box is given in Table 19.4. The person wore their normal indoor clothing and then put on different designs of cleanroom clothing made from the same good quality synthetic fabric.

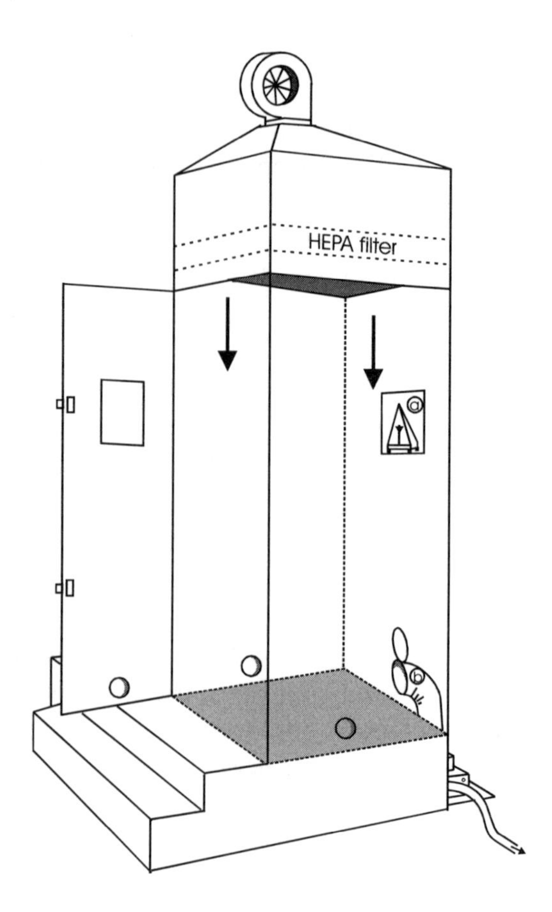

Figure 19.13 Body box: a, metronome; b, bacterial and particle sampler

It is clear from these results that the more the clothing envelops the wearer, the better the result. A surgical-type gown worn over a person's everyday clothing is effective in reducing dispersion, but cannot stop the dispersion coming out from underneath it. A shirt and trouser system is more effective, but air will spill out the open neck and trouser legs. When a coverall with a tuck-in hood and knee-high boots is worn the best result are obtained.

Table 19.4 Effect of design on bacterial dispersal rate (counts per minute)

Own clothes	Gown over own clothes	Open-necked shirt and trousers of good fabric	Cleanroom coverall
610	180	113.9	7.5

19.6.2.2 Comparison of clothing made from different fabrics

A comparison was made of a male volunteer wearing his normal indoor clothing and cleanroom clothing. The volunteer wore either (a) his underpants only, (b) his normal underpants, shirt, trousers, socks and shoes and (c) different types of cleanroom suits with hood, full-length overboots and latex gloves. The different types of cleanroom suits were made from three fabrics. These were:

1. the poor open fabric shown in Figure 19.5 with a pore diameter of about 100 μm;
2. the tighter fabric shown in Figure 19.9 with a pore diameter of about 50 μm;
3. GoreTex fabric made from a membrane sandwiched onto polyester fabric and impermeable to the sizes of particles measured.

A GoreTex suit was also tested with special elasticised closures designed to make an escape of air less likely.

Shown in Table 19.5 is the average number of bacteria dispersed per minute from the male volunteer when he wore different sets of clothing. The greatest dispersion occurred when only underpants were worn, but the addition of another filtration layer, i.e. his shirt and trousers, reduced the rate. However, this would not be paralleled if inert particle counts were measured, unless the clothing was low linting and had good filtration properties. It can also be seen that the poor fabric with large pores reduces bacterial dispersion, but a tight fabric performed even better.

Table 19.5 Bacterial dispersion (counts/min) in relation to fabrics

Underpants	Underpants + shirt + trousers	Open-fabric	Tight fabric	Gore-Tex	GoreTex 'special closures'
1108	487	103	11	27	0.6

As the air permeability increases, the amount of air pumped out of the garments' closures, (i.e. cuffs, neck etc.) increases. The pressure inside a GoreTex suit is many times greater than a garment made of a woven fabric. This is reflected in the fact that a higher dispersion rate than expected was found. However, when a GoreTex garment with special closures to minimise air escape was tested, a further large reduction in bacterial dispersion was achieved. This gave a dispersion rate 170 times less than the open fabric.

The above tests were also carried out to measure dust particles. Shown in Table 19.6 is the particle dispersion per minute.

Table 19.6 Particle dispersion rate per minute in relation to fabric

	Own clothes	Open fabric	Tighter fabric	Gortex	Gortex 'special closures'
Particles ≥ 0.5 μm	4.5×10^6	8.5×10^5	5.0×10^5	8.2×10^5	3.5×10^4
Particles ≥ 5.0 μm	1.2×10^4	3550	3810	2260	74

It is interesting to note the general ineffectiveness of cleanroom clothing in preventing the dispersion of small particles (≥ 0.5 μm). If the 'special closures' GoreTex clothing are excluded, it is seen that cleanroom clothing gave only a small reduction in the dispersion of particles ≥ 0.5 μm (from 10^6/min to 10^5/min). However, these cleanroom garments were much more effective in removing larger (≥ 5.0 μm) particles.

19.7 Static Dissipative Properties of Clothing

The antistatic property of clothing is important in some parts of the clean-room industry, e.g. in the microelectronics industry where electrostatic charges may destroy micro-circuits. As people move around the clean-room, the rubbing of their cleanroom clothing against seats and benches, as well as inner clothing and skin, generates electrostatic charges within the fabric. This static electricity can then discharge to a microcircuit and destroy it. Cleanroom fabrics are therefore manufactured with continuous threads of conducting material built into the fabric. The following tests can be used to choose clothing that minimise electrostatic discharge:

- the measurement of the resistivity, or conductivity;
- the measurement of the voltage decay;
- the measurement of the voltage produced by a moving person when wearing a garment.

Several methods exist for determining the surface resistance of fabrics. The lower the resistance, the better the fabric, as it is assumed that static electricity is more easily conducted away.

The antistatic properties of a fabric may be measured by noting the time it takes for a given static charge to decay from the fabric. This is a better test than measuring conductivity. A known charge is generated on the fabric, and the time for this to reduce to ½ (or 1/10) of its voltage is determined. Times quoted can vary from less than 0.1 second to over 10 minutes, a shorter time indicating a better fabric.

Shown in Table 19.7 are results published by the British Textile Technology Group, comparing the static charge generated by people wearing garments made of two fabrics. The fabrics were identical except that one had antistatic strips (resistivity of 10^6) and the other fabric was without strips (resistivity 10^{13}). A person wearing a garment made from one of these fabrics got up from a chair and their body voltage was measured when they touched a voltmeter. When the person and chair were insulated from earth, a maximum voltage of 3210 volts was obtained from the standard fabric, and 2500 volts from the fabric with the conductive strips. This is not a very large benefit. However, if the chair was earthed and conductive footwear worn, substantially better results were obtained (see Table 19.6). These results emphasise the need for earthing the chair, the person and the clothing. They also show the limitations of conductive strips in fabrics. Not investigated was the effect of electrically connecting the various items of fabric in a garment. Where the various parts of the garment are conventionally stitched together the conduction of electrostatic charge is poor. This can be substantially improved if the garment parts are electrically connected.

Table 19.7 Body voltage with and without antistatic strips

	Antistatic strips	No strips
Resistivity (ohms)	10^6	10^{13}
Maximum body voltage - insulated leather chair	2500V	3210V
Maximum body voltage - earthed; leather chair; conductive footwear	160V	760 V

Acknowledgements

Figure 19.3 is reproduced by permission of the Science Photo Library. Figure 19.6 is reproduced by permission of St John's Institute of Dermatology. Figures 19.7 and 19.8 are reproduced by permission of Contamination Control Apparel. Figure 19.10 is reproduced by permission of C W Berndt. Figure 19.11 is reproduced by permission of Fishers Services. Tables 19.1, 19.2 and 19.3 are compiled from information made available by permission of the Institute of Environmental Sciences and Technology.

20

Cleanroom Masks and Gloves

20.1 Cleanroom Masks

People expel large numbers of saliva droplets from their mouth when sneezing, coughing and talking. These droplets contain salts and bacteria, and it is necessary to prevent them causing contamination in the cleanroom. Wearing a mask over the face normally does this.

The dispersion of droplets and the means of controlling dispersion are discussed below.

20.1.1 Dispersion from the mouth

Shown in Table 20.1 are typical numbers of particles and microbe-carrying particles that are dispersed by sneezing, coughing and speaking loudly. The number of particles produced by breathing is not reported but is low and difficult to ascertain accurately.

Table 20.1 Number of inert and microbe-carrying particles emitted by a person

	Inert particles	Microbe-carrying particles
One sneeze	1 000 000	39 000
One cough	5000	700
Loud speaking (100 words)	250	40

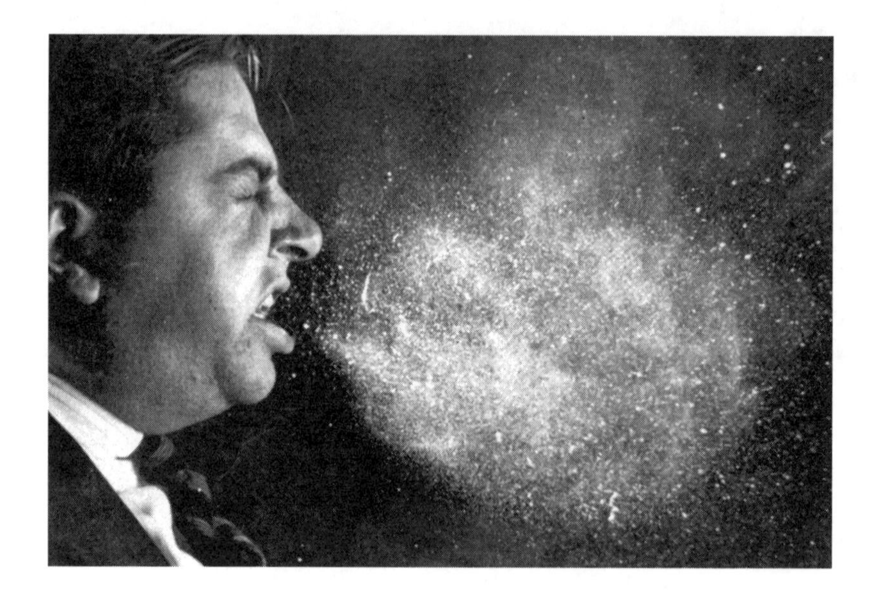

Figure 20.1 Particles emitted during a sneeze

Figure 20.1 shows droplets produced by a sneeze frozen in mid air by high-speed photography. Figure 20.2 shows the lower number of droplets that are produced by pronouncing the letter 'f'.

Saliva particles and droplets dispersed from the mouth vary in diameter from about 1 μm to about 2000 μm; 95% of them lie being between 2 and 100 μm, with an average size of about 50 μm. Although the count of bacteria in saliva is normally over 10^7 bacteria per ml, not all of the emitted particles will contain bacteria.

What happens to these expelled droplets and particles depends on their size and hence their rate of drying and settling. If the particles are large, their rate of settling caused by gravitational forces is high, and they will fall quickly and not have time to dry. Small particles will not fall quickly, but will dry and pass into the air circulation of the cleanroom.

The time it takes for particles of water to deposit by gravity can be calculated. A 100 μm particle will drop 1 metre in about 3 seconds, but a 10 μm particle takes about 5 minutes. It is also possible to calculate the drying time. Particles of water 1000 μm in diameter will take about 3 minutes to evaporate, a 200 μm particle will take 7 seconds, a 100 μm particle about 1.6 seconds and a 50 μm particle about 0.4 seconds. It can be calculated that particles have to be less than about 200 μm if they are to dry before they drop a distance of one metre. It therefore follows that some very large droplets of saliva can drop onto products if a facemask is not used.

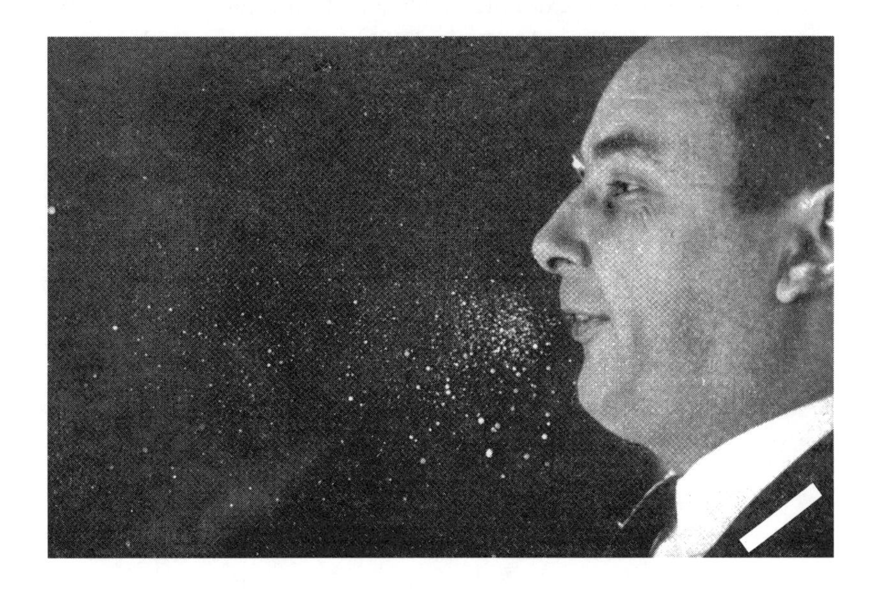

Figure 20.2 Particles emitted when pronouncing the letter 'f'

Because of the small amount of dissolved material in saliva, the evaporation of water from the drops of expelled saliva reduces the droplets to about one-quarter to one-seventh of their size. These dried particles, known as droplet nuclei, pass into the air circulation in the room.

Many of the particles expelled from the mouth are of sufficient size and inertia to be projected onto the inner surface of a face mask, where they will be easily stopped and retained by a layer of fabric. Efficiencies of over 95% for particles expelled from the mouth are usually obtained by most masks. A loss in efficiency is caused by particles passing round the side of the mask, and much of this is due to small particles (reported to be $< 3\mu m$ in the dry state).

20.1.2 Face masks

Masks vary in design, but all are made of some type of material placed in front of the mouth and nose so that when a person is talking, coughing, sneezing or snorting, the particles expelled are impacted against it, or remove by filtration. A common form of mask is the surgical-style with straps and loops, a typical example being shown in Figure 20.3. The type shown is a disposable surgical-type made from a non-woven fabric and is thrown away when exiting the cleanroom.

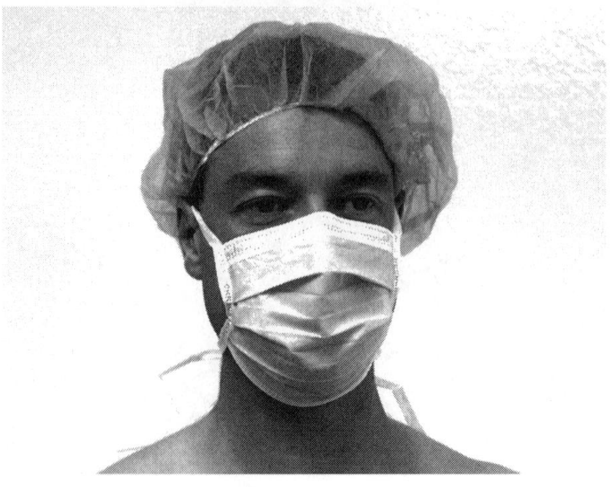

Figure 20.3 Disposable surgical-type face mask

Consideration should be made of the pressure drop across the mask fabric. Manufacturers can produce masks that have very high filtration efficiency against small particles. However, this high filtration efficiency may be unnecessary, because of the relatively large size of the expelled droplets and can give a high-pressure drop across the mask that causes the generated particles to be forced round the outside of the mask. This higher pressure can be reduced by the use of masks with a larger surface area of material.

Another type of mask is the 'veil' or 'yashmak' type, one of this type being exposed to show its shape in Figure 20.4. The normal way it is worn is shown in Figure 20.5.

Veils can be snapped into hoods, or permanently sewn into the hood at manufacture. Care should be taken to select a material and style that not only controls the risk from emissions from the mouth, but which is acceptable to personnel.

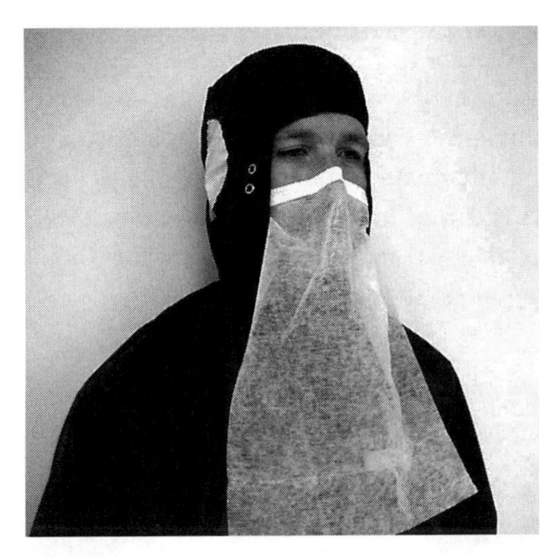

Figure 20.4 Veil or yashmak- type mask shown outside the hood

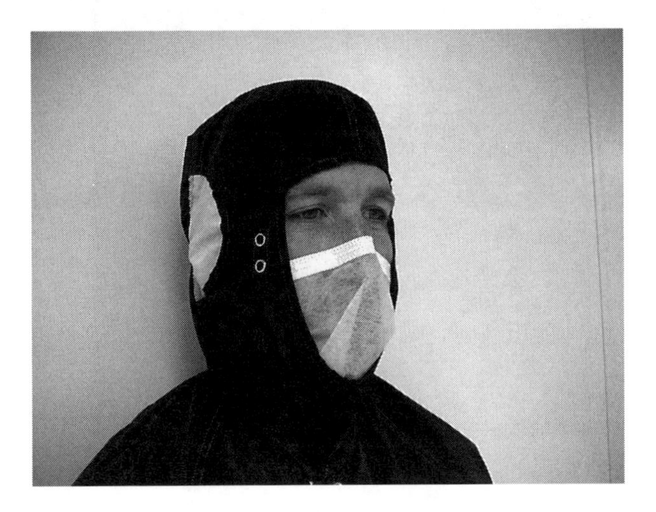

Figure 20.5 Veil or yashmak type mask as normally worn

Glasses or goggles can provide an additional barrier to skin flakes, eyebrow hair and eyelashes and keep them from falling onto critical surfaces (see Figure 17.3 in Chapter 17).

20.1.3 Powered exhaust headgear

Several designs of powered exhaust headgear are available. These provide a barrier to contamination coming from the head, as well as the mouth; they also remove contamination pumped out of the neck closure of the garment. The exhaust from the helmet and face-shield is provided with a filtered exhaust system so that contamination does not escape into the cleanroom. An example is shown in Figure 20.6.

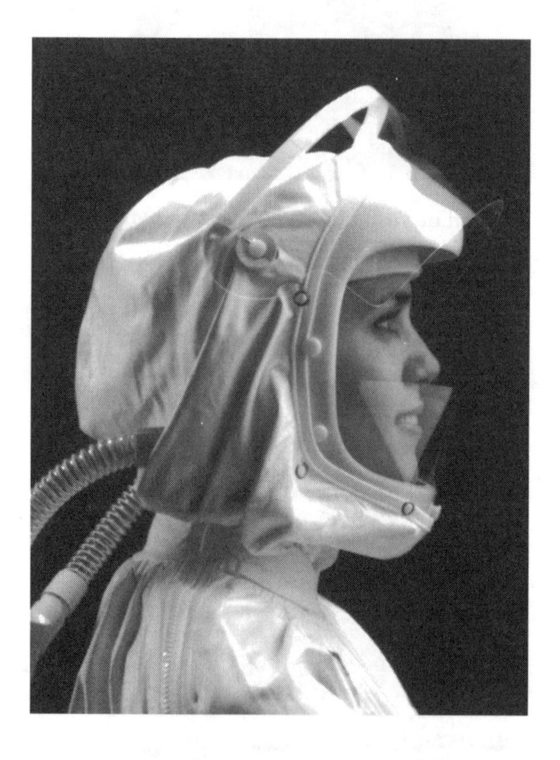

Figure 20.6 Powered exhaust helmet

20.2 Cleanroom Gloves

20.2.1 Hand contamination and gloves

People's hands have millions of skin particles and bacteria on them, as well as surface oils and salts. To prevent this being transferred onto contamination sensitive products, gloves should be worn.

There are two types of gloves associated with cleanrooms. Knitted or woven gloves are used for lower classes, i.e. ISO Class 7 (Class 10,000) and poorer areas, as well as undergloves. The knit or weave should be tight and a number of loose threads minimised. This type of glove is not discussed further. Barrier gloves, which have a continuous thin membrane covering the whole hand are used in the majority of cleanrooms.

There are a number of problems associated with cleanroom gloves. Their surface may not be sufficiently free of contamination, as they are not usually manufactured in a cleanroom; they therefore require cleaning before being used. They should thus be selected with regard to their surface contamination and, depending on the type of use, be free of particles, oils, chemicals or micro-organisms. Gloves can be punctured during use, and this allows contamination to pass out. For example, it has been shown that the number of bacteria coming through a glove when it was punctured to give a 1mm hole was 7000 from an unwashed hand, and 2000 from a washed hand.

Gloves may be required in some cleanrooms to prevent dangerous chemicals, usually acids or solvents, attacking the operator's hands. An example of this problem is the use of acids in the wet-etch step in semiconductor manufacturing. This should be borne in mind when the glove is chosen, as thicker and stronger gloves are required.

Some operator's skin is allergic to the materials that gloves are made from. Accelerators in latex, nitrile and neoprene gloves, and the protein in latex, can cause skin irritations. Hypoallergenic gloves, or inner fabric liners, should be worn to minimise this effect.

Other glove properties that should be considered when choosing a glove are chemical resistance and compatibility, electrostatic discharge properties, surface ion contribution when wet, contact transfer, barrier integrity, permeability to liquids, heat resistance and outgassing.

20.2.2 Glove manufacturing process

Gloves are generally manufactured by dipping a 'former', the shape of a hand, into molten or liquid glove material. Formers are usually made of porcelain or stainless steel. The former is removed from the molten or liquid material, and a layer of material allowed to set to form a glove. The glove is then stripped from the former. To allow the gloves to be removed from the former without damage, a release agent is normally employed on the former's surface. When removed, the release agent will contaminate the outside of the glove. Release agents are a problem in cleanrooms, and hence cleanroom gloves differ from domestic ones in that the release agent is kept to a minimum. Gloves are also washed with a view to removing the release agent and any other additives added to the dipping medium. An example of this is the use of Magnesium silicate as a release agent in latex gloves made for domestic use. If the Magnesium silicate is replaced with Calcium carbonate, this powder can be removed from the surface by a mild acid wash. Another way of dealing with the release agent is during stripping. When the gloves are stripped from the former they are 'inside-out', and they may then be turned 'outside-out' to offset the release agent problem.

Glove formulations used in manufacturing non-cleanroom gloves can contain about 15 additives, and a number of these can cause contamination in cleanrooms. Cleanroom gloves may differ from those used domestically by minimising, or not using, some of these chemicals.

When stripped from the formers, latex gloves are 'sticky'. To correct this, latex gloves are washed in a chlorine bath. The free chlorine combines chemically with the latex chemical bonds and lead to a 'case-hardening' of the surface of the glove, which prevents them sticking to each other. This washing also helps to clean to the gloves.

20.2.3 Types of gloves

20.2.3.1 Polyvinyl chloride (PVC) gloves

These plastic gloves are also known as vinyl gloves and are popular in electronic cleanrooms. This type of glove cannot be satisfactorily sterilised, and are therefore not used in bioclean rooms. They are available in normal and long-sleeve length, and should preferably be long enough to cover the cuff of the garment sleeve. Consideration should be made of the fact that plasticisers make up almost 50% of a vinyl glove. Plasticisers come from the same group of chemicals used to test the integrity of air filters, i.e. phthalates. This material is necessary to make the glove pliable, and also has the advantage of giving the gloves some antistatic properties. However, it can also causes contamination problem from outgassing and contact transfer onto surfaces.

20.2.3.2 Latex Gloves

This is the type used by surgeons, and the 'particle-free' type is now used in cleanrooms. Latex gloves can be produced 'powder-free', and those gloves that are washed further by use of filtered, deionised water are often used in ISO Class 4 (Class 10) or ISO Class 3 (Class 1) cleanrooms.

They have good chemical resistance, giving protection against most weak acids and bases, and alcohols, as well as having a fairly good resistance against aldehydes and ketones. They are slightly more expensive to buy than the PVC type, but cheaper than any other polymer. They can be sterilised. Because of their elasticity, the glove can securely incorporate the cuff of a garment under the sleeve.

20.2.3.3 Other Polymer Gloves

Polythene gloves are used in cleanrooms and have the advantage of being free of oils and additives, as well as resistant to puncturing. They are not resistant to aliphatic solvents. The main drawback of this glove type is that they are constructed from float sheets and the seams are welded. Manual dexterity is reduced with these gloves.

Neoprene and nitrile gloves are chemically similar to latex gloves, but have the advantage of having a better resistance to solvents than latex gloves. They are slightly more expensive than latex.

Polyurethane gloves are strong, very thin, quite inflexible, and expensive. They may be manufactured with microporous material for better comfort, or with carbon in the formulation which makes them conductive.

PVA gloves are resistant to strong acids and solvents, but not water in which they are soluble. They are expensive.

Gore-Tex gloves have welded seams and are hypoallergenic. They are breathable because of their porous membrane. They are expensive.

Special gloves are used in cleanrooms for heat resistance or insulation and usually made from polymers of silicone, or Kevlar. They are generally not made for cleanroom use and, when used in cleanrooms, they should be cleaned thoroughly and their contact with contamination-sensitive material minimised. Kevlar gloves have a special problem because of their fibrous nature.

Other polymers, such a butyl rubber, are occasionally used to make gloves for use in cleanrooms. Careful evaluation of the cleanliness of these products must be done before accepting them for use.

20.2.4 Testing of Gloves

Information on the properties of gloves and methods used to test gloves is given in the Institute of Environmental Sciences Recommended Practice, RP CC005. Tests for surface cleanliness include the measurement of particles, non-volatile residues and ions.

Particle counting involves submerging a sample in a quantity of particle-free water, and shaking on an orbital shaker for a given time. The water from the sample is then analysed for particles, either by use of a liquid particle counter, or microscopically.

Measurement of the non-volatile residue involves submerging a sample in a suitable solvent, at a given temperature, for a given period of time. The sample is removed and the weight of the residue from the evaporated solvent measured. Ionic content is measured by submerging a sample in deionised water for a period of time then measuring the ion content of the water.

Other tests include chemical resistance and compatibility; strength and accelerated ageing of the barrier material; static charge; permeability resistance to liquids; contact transfer; outgassing, and heat resistance. These are detailed in IEST -RP-CC005.

It may be necessary to ensure that gloves are not punctured after use. There are simple methods available for checking tears and holes in gloves. The used glove can be filled with water and checked for leaks. The glove can also be blown up with air (by mouth is sufficient), closed at the cuff, and squeezed; any leaks can be found by passing the glove close to the cheek.

Acknowledgements

Figures 20.1 and 20.2 are reproduced by permission of the American Association for the Advancement of Science. I should like to thank Douglas Fraser of the Protein Fractionation Clinic for posing for the photograph for Figure 20.3 and Michael Perry of Analog Devices for posing for the photographs in Figures 20.4 and 20.5. Figure 20.6 is reproduced by permission of Pentagon Technologies.

21

Cleaning a Cleanroom

21.1 Why a Cleanroom Must be Cleaned

Cleanrooms are used to protect the products of many industries from contamination. Millions of pounds or dollars, as well as years of effort, can be put into designing and constructing a cleanroom, but little thought and effort may go into keeping the room clean.

It may be asked, 'Why does a cleanroom need to be cleaned. Is it not supplied with large quantities of particle and bacterial-free air, and do not workers wear special cleanroom clothing to prevent dispersion of contamination'? In fact, cleanroom clothing, as has been discussed in Chapter 19, does not stop dispersion and a person can disperse, when wearing cleanroom clothing, over 100 000 particles ≥ 0.5 μm and over 10 000 particles ≥ 5.0 μm. Machines also disperse millions of particles. Many of the larger particles will easily settle, by gravity, onto horizontal surfaces. Other smaller particles are thrown from the air stream, or deposited by Brownian motion, onto surfaces. Dirt can also be brought into a cleanroom through foot-borne transfer.

Cleanrooms surfaces get dirty and must be cleaned. If they are not, contamination is transmitted to the product when it comes into contact with the dirty surfaces; it can also be transferred by personnel touching a cleanroom surface and then the product. Cleanrooms can appear to be clean but can, in terms of cleanroom requirements, be very dirty. The human eye will not see a particle much smaller than 50 μm. Small particles will eventually be seen when their concentration builds up and agglomeration occurs. When this happens, a cleanroom is long past being acceptably clean.

People can also disperse hundreds, or thousands, of microbe-carrying particles per minute. Because these micro-organisms are carried on skin cells, or fragments of skin cells, their average equivalent diameter is between 10 μm and 20 μm. These settle easily, by gravity, onto surfaces in the room. In cleanrooms, such as those used by the healthcare industry, the room must be disinfected to kill the micro-organisms.

21.2 Cleaning Methods and the Physics of Cleaning Surfaces

The main force that holds particles to cleanroom surfaces is the London-van der Waal's force, this being an inter-molecular force. Electrostatic forces can also attract particles to a surface. The importance of electrostatic forces will vary between cleanrooms, and depends on the type of materials used within the cleanroom. A third force can arise after wet cleaning. Particles that are left behind will dry on the surface, and may adhere to it through a bridge of material that has dried out from the liquid left behind.

If aqueous solutions are used for cleaning then particles that are water-soluble will be dissolved. If solvents such as alcohols are used, then organic materials are dissolved; these particles can then be removed in solution. However, the majority of particles found in a cleanroom cannot be dissolved, and the adhesive force that holds particles to a surface must be overcome. Immersing the particle in a liquid, as occurs in wet pick-up vacuuming, damp wiping or mopping, may dissolve the particle bridge left after drying. If an aqueous-based detergent is used then the London-van der Waal's force and electrostatic forces can be reduced or eliminated. The particle can then be pushed or drawn off from a surface by wiping, mopping or vacuuming.

The methods that are generally used for cleaning a cleanroom, are:

- Vacuuming (wet or dry)
- Wet wiping (mopping or damp wiping)
- Picking-up with a tacky roller.

The efficiency of these cleaning methods depends on the surface being wiped. If the surface finish is rough or pitted then it is more difficult to remove particles situated within these surface blemishes. Thus it is necessary, as discussed in Chapter 8, that the inner surfaces in a cleanroom should be smooth.

21.2.1 Vacuuming

There are two types of vacuuming used to clean cleanrooms: dry and wet. Dry vacuuming depends on a jet of air moving towards the vacuum nozzle and overcoming the adhesion forces of particles to the surface, and hence detaching them from a surface. However, an air velocity cannot be generated that is sufficient to remove small particles.

Figure 21.1 is a graph of results I obtained to show the efficiency of dry vacuuming against different sizes of sand particles on a glass surface.

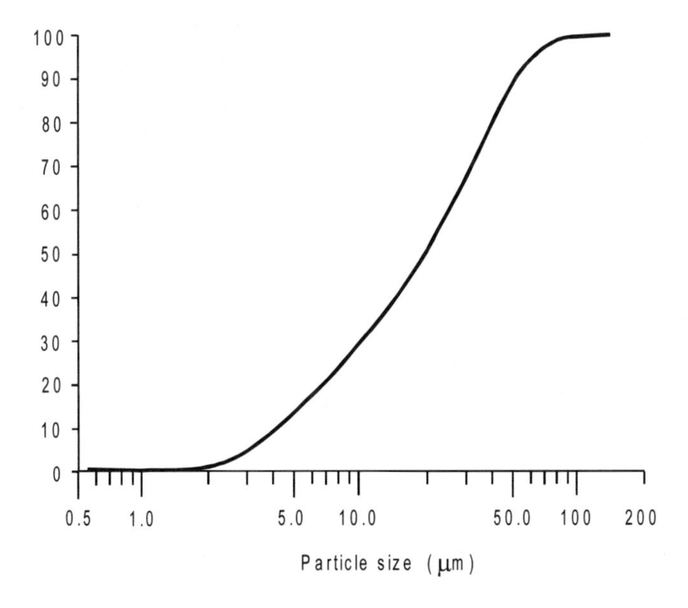

Figure 21.1 Efficiency of dry vacuuming

A nozzle of an industrial vacuum was pushed along a surface covered with particles. It may be seen that most of the particles over 100 μm are removed, but smaller particles are inefficiently removed, and at a size of 10 μm only about 25% are removed. This experiment shows that the majority of particles on surfaces are not removed by dry vacuuming, and domestic experience confirms this. How many people would be content to only vacuum a vinyl floor? A light-coloured kitchen floor would, in a very short time, be in an unacceptable condition.

Water and solvents have much higher viscosity than air, so that the drag forces exerted by liquids on a surface particle are very much greater. Therefore, if a wet pick-up vacuum system is used, the additional drag forces will substantially increase the collection efficiency.

21.2.2 Wet wiping

Wet wiping, with wipers or mops, can efficiently clean cleanroom surfaces. The liquid used allows some of the particle-to-surface bonds to be broken and particles to float off. This is especially true if a surfactant is used. However, many particles still adhere to the surface, and the mop or wiper's fibres are necessary to push and detach the particles. The particles that are removed are retained in the wiper. A damp wiper is more efficient than a dry one, as the drag forces in the aqueous solution or solvent are much greater.

Some wipers and mops are more efficient than others. As they work by pushing and dragging particles, a wiper or mop made from a fine fibrous material will be more efficient that a solid block of material.

21.2.3 Tacky rollers

The particle removal efficiency of 'tacky' rollers is dependent on the strength of the adhesive force of the roller's surface. The greater this force, the more particles that are removed. Other factors, such as the surface softness of the roller, which allows better contact with the particle's surface, will also influence the removal efficiency.

21.3 Implements Used to Clean Cleanrooms

The implements used in cleanrooms have a similarity to those used in cleaning the home. However, there are important differences. For example, a dry brush should never be used to sweep a cleanroom. I found that they can produce over 50 million particles ≥ 0.5 μm per minute. String mops are not much better, as they can produce almost 20 million particles ≥ 0.5 μm per minute.

21.3.2 Dry and wet vacuum systems

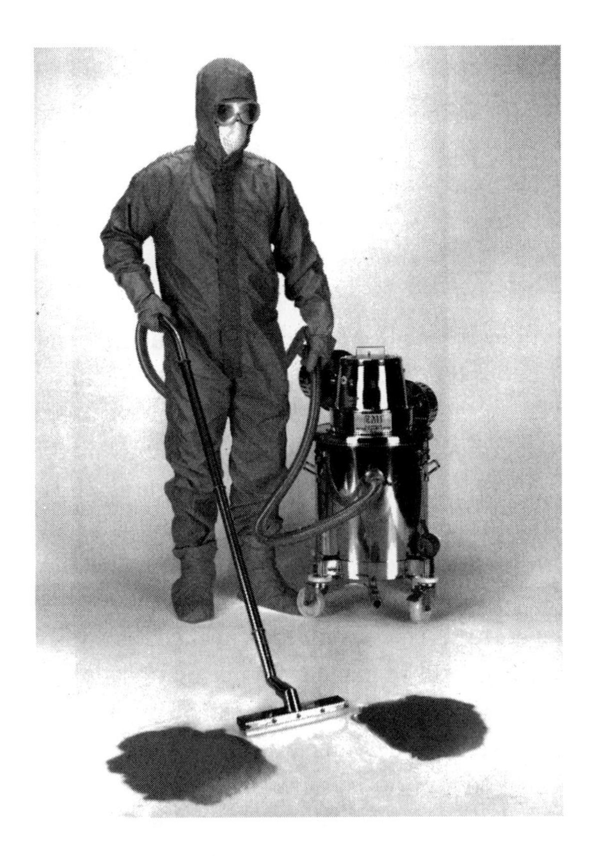

Figure 21.2 Vacuum system being used in its wet pick-up mode

Dry vacuuming is a popular method of cleaning because it is relatively inexpensive and, because no cleaning liquids are needed, no contaminants are introduced into the cleanroom. However, unfiltered exhaust-air must not pass into the cleanroom. This is achieved by using either an external central-vacuum source, or providing a portable vacuum's exhaust air with a HEPA or ULPA filter. This filter must be placed after the motor to ensure that no particles from the motor are dispersed into the room.

A wet vacuum or 'pick-up' system is more efficient than a dry vacuum system because of the additional drag forces from the liquid used. It is also generally more efficient than a mopping method, as there is less liquid left to dry on the floor, and hence contaminate it; this also means that the floor will also dry quicker. Figure 21.2 shows a cleanroom vacuum system being used in its wet pick-up mode to clean a cleanroom floor. Wet pick-up systems are used on conventionally ventilated cleanroom floors, but may not be suitable for the pass-though type of floor used in the vertical unidirectional system.

21.3.2 Mopping systems

Cleanrooms are often cleaned with a mop and bucket. Household string mops should not be used as they contribute a large amount of contamination. Squeezy-type sponge and other synthetic mops used in the home contribute less contamination when new, but break up through use.

Two types of cleanroom mops are shown in Figures 21.3 and 21.4. The cleaning surfaces of these mops are made from materials that do not easily break up. This can be made from a PVA or polyurethane open-pore foam, or a fabric such as polyester. The compatibility of the material to sterilisation, disinfectants and solvents should be checked, as some materials are not suitable. Buckets should be made from plastic or stainless steel.

A cleanroom can be cleaned and disinfected by use of a mop and a bucket containing water with detergent, or disinfectant. However, the level of cleanliness achieved by this system may not be sufficient for some cleanrooms, as the dirt taken from the floor is rinsed out into the bucket and reapplied to the floor. Experience in the home tells us that it does not take long before the detergent solution is dirty and the floor is not being cleaned properly.

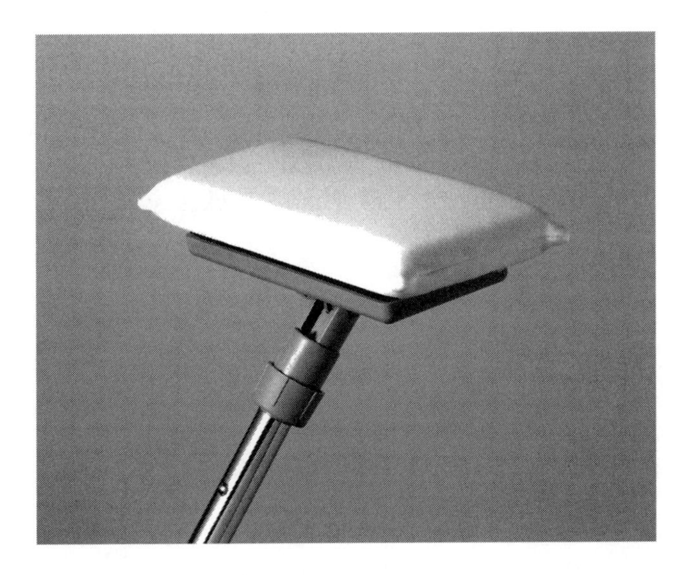

Figure 21.3 Cleanroom mop suitable for cleaning surfaces such as walls

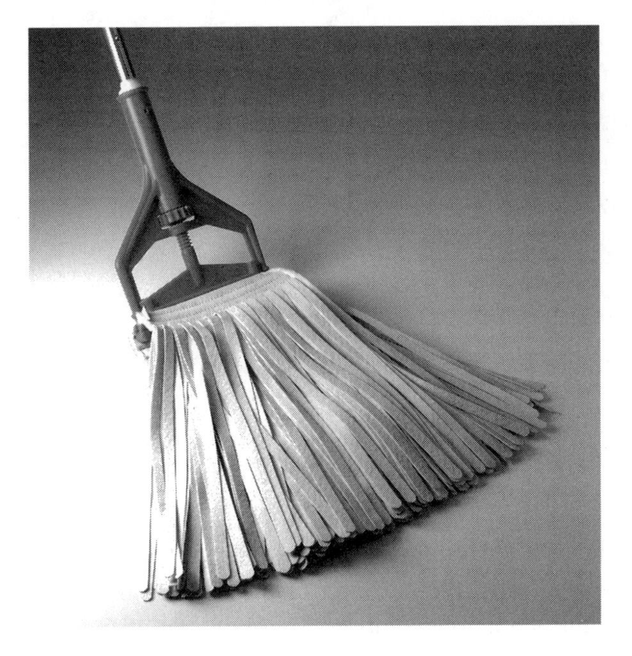

Figure 21.4 Cleanrooms mop suitable for floors

When disinfectants are used, especially chlorine-based ones, the soil contamination may neutralise the disinfectant's effectiveness. Continual changing of the solution in the bucket overcomes this problem, but a substantial improvement can also be made by use of a '2 or 3-bucket' system. Figure 21.5 is a photograph of 2-bucket and 3-bucket' systems.

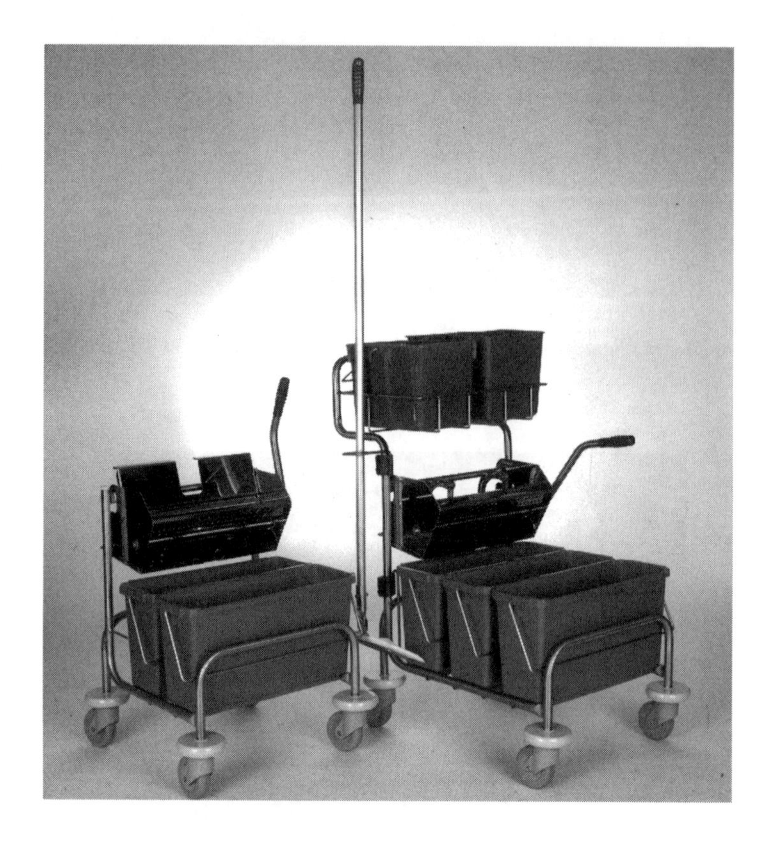

Figure 21.5 Two and three bucket systems

Figure 21.6 shows a diagram of a method I suggest for the 2- or 3- bucket system. As can be seen, the cleaning or disinfection starts with the mop being dipped into the active solution. The mop can, if thought necessary, be squeezed free of excess liquid. The liquid is then spread onto the floor and the floor wiped, or disinfected (stage 1). The mop is then wrung free of much of the dirty water collected in the mop (stage 2), dipped, and rinsed in the clean water (stage 3). The mop is again wrung free of excess liquid (stage 4) dipped into the active solution (stage 5), and is then ready to carry out the same cycle again (stage 1).

If a 2-bucket system is used, one bucket is filled with active solution and the other with clean water, although an alternative is to use the second bucket for collecting waste liquid. However, the 2-bucket system is not as efficient as the 3-bucket system.

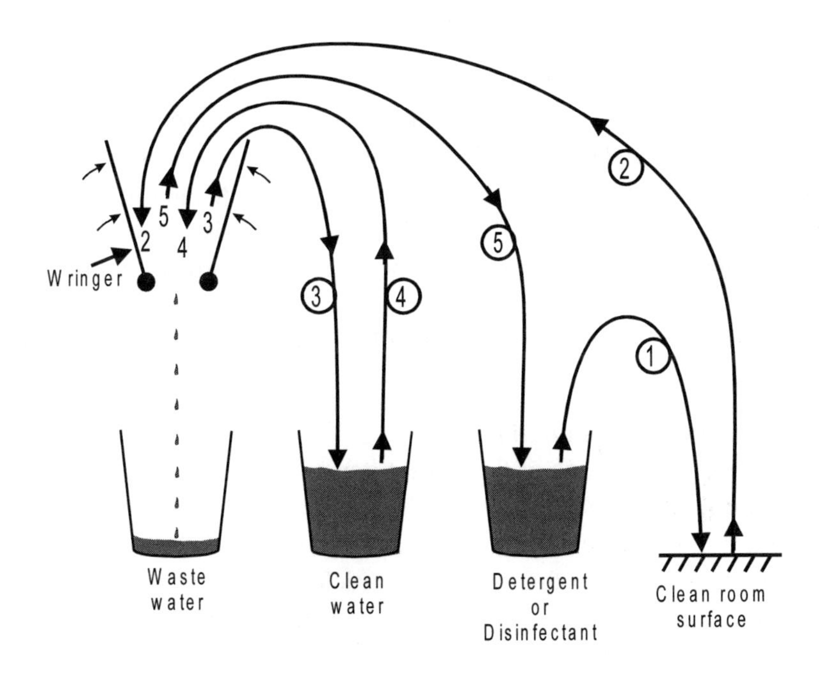

Figure 21.6 How to use a three-bucket mopping system

21.3.3 Wipers

Wipers are dampened with a detergent or disinfectant solution and used in cleanrooms to wipe surfaces and remove contamination. They are also used to wipe contamination from products produced in the room and used dry to mop-up liquids that may have been spilled. Normal household wipers are not acceptable in cleanrooms as they have a high concentration of particle, fibre and chemical contamination that is left on the surfaces they clean.

The choice of wipers depends on the contamination problems in the cleanroom. There is no perfect wiper that removes all contamination from a surface; the selection of a wiper is a compromise. Knowing the use the wiper has to be put to, the importance attached to its properties, and the cash available, the best wiper can be selected for the job. The properties of wipers that should be considered are as follows.

21.3.3.1 Sorbency

Sorbency is an important property of wipers. Wipers are often used to mop up a spillage and other similar tasks. It is therefore necessary to know the wiper's sorbency; both its capacity (the amount of liquid it can sorb) and its rate (how fast it can sorb liquid). This property is also important in terms of contamination control, as a wiper with good sorbency will ensure that less contamination is left on the surface than one with poor sorbency; if a cleanroom surface is wiped and little liquid left, then there will be fewer particles left.

21.3.3.2 Wiper contamination

Cleanroom wipers are one of the dirtiest items in a cleanroom. Compared to wipers used in the home they are clean, but a single wiper can contain many times more particles than all the air in the room. It is therefore necessary to choose a wiper that is low in particles. Attention should also be paid to the edges of the wiper as raw edges can contribute to fibre and particle contamination.

When a wiper is wetted, any material within the wiper that is soluble will dissolve. This may then be transferred onto the surface being wiped. Materials that can be extracted by water, or solvents, are known as 'extractables'. Extractables of particular interest in the semiconductor industry are metallic ions. When this is important the amount and type of extractables in a wiper can be used to determine the best wiper for the job.

21.3.3.3 Other properties of wipers
Other properties that should be considered are:

- textile strength
- abrasion resistance
- static (or antistatic) properties
- sterility.

All of the above properties of wipers can be evaluated by the tests suggested in the IEST Recommended Practice RP CC004.

21.3.4 Tacky rollers

Tacky rollers are similar in size and shape to paint rollers used in the home, but they have a tacky material around the outside of the roller. An example of a tacky roller is shown in Figure 21.7.

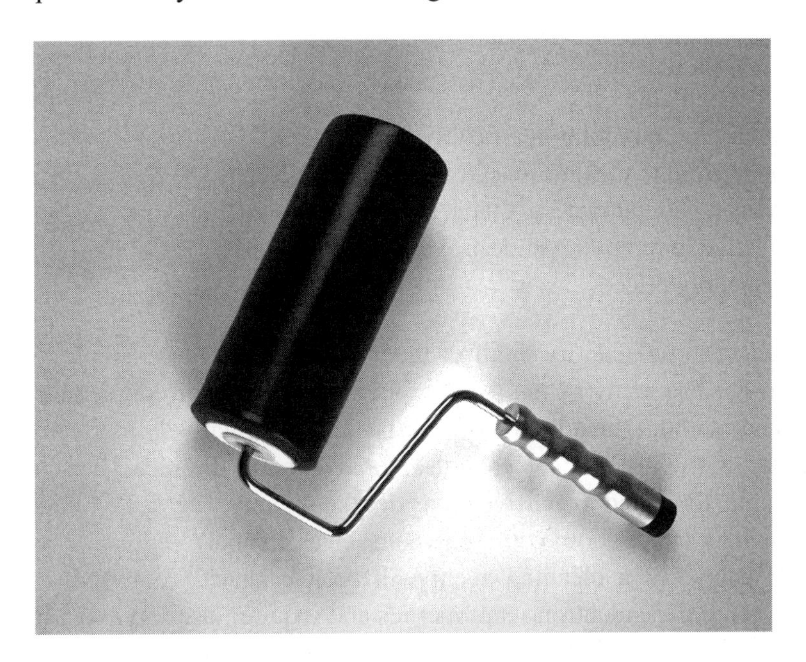

Figure 21.7 Tacky roller

The roller is rolled over a cleanroom surface and particles adhere to the roller's tacky surface.

21.3.5 Floor scrubbing systems

Floor scrubbing machines that use rotary brushes are available for cleanroom use. The machine has a skirt around the outside of the brushes and an exhaust system that removes particles produced by brushing the floor. A high efficiency filter then filters this exhaust.

21.4 Liquids Used in Cleaning Cleanrooms

21.4.1 Cleaning liquids

The ideal cleaning solution for a cleanroom is one that has the following properties:

- non-toxic to people
- non-flammable
- fast drying, but not unreasonably so
- not harmful to cleanroom surfaces
- leaves no contamination that is harmful to the product
- effective in removing undesirable contamination
- reasonably priced.

No product is satisfactory in all of the above aspects. For example, ultra-clean water has many of the listed properties but can corrode certain surfaces and, without the addition of a surfactant, it is relatively ineffective in cleaning. Some organic solvents also come close to the ideal, but can be flammable, toxic and expensive (consider the toxicity, fire danger and cost of cleaning a whole room with a solvent such as ethanol).

The choice of a cleaning agent will be a balanced compromise, the choice being dependent on its properties and required use. To assist in the correct choice, knowledge of the properties of the cleaning solution must be considered.

The toxicity, flammability and boiling point properties of various solvents are available from the suppliers of solvents, and these will assist in the choice of a suitable solvent. Also available is information on the effect solvents have on materials. Important in the context of cleaning cleanrooms is its effect on plastics, some of which are very vulnerable to solvents.

Because of their toxicity and flammability it is difficult to find a good choice of solvent. The demise of CFCs because of environmental problems has added to the problem. Alcohols are often used, especially when combined with water to reduce the flammability of the alcohol and increase their disinfection properties.

Cleaning is often carried out by water containing a surfactant. However, cleaning agents in their household form are often combined with chemicals such as perfumes, sodium chloride, sodium carbonate, sodium meta silicate, tetra-potassium pyro-phosphate, formaldehyde, etc., and the choice of such surfactants may be a mistake. Cleaning agents which are chemically less reactive are best.

Surfactants have a hydrocarbon water-repellent (hydrophobic) group and a water-attracting (hydrophilic) group. They can therefore be divided into four groups, depending on whether the hydrophobic part of the molecule is anionic, cationic, amphoteric or non-ionic. These are illustrated in Figure 20.8.

The surfactant of choice for cleaning a cleanroom is usually non-ionic, as these are the least reactive of the four types of surfactant and do not contain metallic ions. Anionic surfactants usually contain metallic ions (usually sodium), but it is possible to manufacture them with organic bases and hence avoid the problem of metallic ions. These anionic compounds will, however, still be reactive.

Finally, some thought must be given to particle contamination. When the detergent solution or organic solvent dries, unacceptable particle contamination must not result. These solutions must be therefore free of particles of significant size. This is particularly important in critical areas close to the production points, e.g. clean benches, but of less significance in general areas away from the production, e.g. walls, doors and floors.

(1) Anionic, e.g. Sodium dodecyl sulphate

$$CH_3CH_2(CH_2)_9CH_2\ O\ SO_3^{(-)}Na^{(+)}$$

(2) Cationic, e.g. Benzylalkonium chloride

$$CH_2—\overset{\displaystyle CH3}{\underset{\displaystyle CH3}{N^{(+)}}}—C_n\,H_{2n+1}\ C1^{(-)}$$

(3) Amphoteric, e.g. Alkyldimethylbetaine

$$R—\overset{\displaystyle CH3}{\underset{\displaystyle CH3}{N^{(+)}}}—CH_2\ COO^{(-)}$$

(4) Non-ionic, e.g. Dodecylalcohol ethoxylate

$$CH_3(CH_2)_{10}CH_2(OCH_2CH_2)_n\ OH$$

Figure 21.8 Surfactant compounds

21.4.2 Disinfectants

Disinfectants are used in bioclean rooms to kill micro-organisms on surfaces. Similar problems to those found in cleaning solutions exist with disinfectants, and some that are very efficient in killing micro-organisms may not be the product of choice in a cleanroom. It is very difficult to produce a disinfectant that is highly toxic to a microbial cell but not the human cell. It is generally found that these two properties go hand-in-hand and the few disinfectants that are effective against microbes, but not toxic, are expensive. It may be useful to select the expensive, least-toxic, solutions for around the critical area where the product sits, but to use less expensive chemicals in general areas such as floors that are away from the product.

Table 21.1 summarises some of the properties of commonly used disinfectants. It may be seen from this table that there is no perfect disinfectant. Generally speaking, phenols, pine oils and chlorine-release compounds are less suitable in critical cleanroom areas because of their toxic properties, and iodophors because of their corrosive and staining properties. However, this statement is a general one, as each of the categories in the table contain a spectrum of activity that is greater or lower than indicated, and both phenols and chlorine-releasing compounds are used successfully in cleanrooms. Chlorine-release compounds are a particular problem. They will kill spores, which are generally not killed by other acceptable disinfectants. Therefore, despite being toxic and corrosive, they are used in cleanrooms. Quaternary ammonium compounds (Quats), or proprietary disinfectants synthesised to optimise toxicity and disinfection, appear to have fewer problems.

Table 21.1 Properties of disinfectants

	Bactericidal effect				**Other properties**				
Type of Disinfectant:	Gram +ve	Gram -ve	Spores	Fungi	Corrosive	Stain	Toxic	Active in soil	Cost
Alcohols	+++	+++	—	++	No	No	No	Yes	+++
Proprietary eg chlorhexidine	+++	+++	—	+	No	No	No	Yes	+++
Quats	+++	+	—	++	Yes/No	No	No	Yes	++
Iodophors	+++	+++	+	++	Yes	Yes	No	Yes	++
Chlorine type	+++	+++	+++	+++	Yes	Yes	Yes	No	+
Phenols	++	+	—	—	No	No	Yes	Yes	+
Pine oils	+	+	—	—	No	No	No	Yes	+

Quats = Quaternary ammonium compounds

Alcohols are suitable for cleanroom use as they have good bactericidal properties and evaporate to leave practically no residue. The use of 60% or 70% ethanol in water, or 70–100% iso-propanol, is particularly recommended at the point of production, where a minimal carry-over of chemicals is desirable. Incorporation of chlorhexidine, or a similar disinfectant, into the alcohol will increase its effectiveness as a bactericide. The use of a disinfectant such as an alcohol, or an alcohol combined with a proprietary bactericide should be confined, by reasons of expense and fire risk, to the critical area. An aqueous solution of quaternary ammonium compounds, or a phenolic compound, could be used to disinfect the rest of the cleanroom.

Washing surfaces with a simple detergent solution that is free from disinfectant is an effective way of removing most of the micro-organisms on hard surfaces (over 80% efficient). However, the addition of disinfectants will reduce the microbial counts by over 90%, and will be necessary to prevent bacteria growing in the washing materials and cleaning solutions left in buckets. If this is not done, subsequent cleaning will spread the bacteria around the cleanroom.

21.5 How Should a Cleanroom be Cleaned?

The methods used to clean cleanrooms will vary according to the standard of cleanliness of the room and its layout. It is therefore necessary to tailor the cleaning method to the cleanroom. The following information may assist this. It is also useful to consult the IEST RP CC018: 'Cleanroom housekeeping – operating and monitoring procedures'.

21.5.1 General points

The following general points should be considered when developing a cleaning method:

- If you can see any dirt in a cleanroom it is neither a *clean room* nor a *cleanroom* and must be cleaned.
- It must be explained to those cleaning the room that they are removing particles or micro-organisms that cannot be seen. Although the cleanroom may look clean it still requires thorough and systematic cleaning.

- Cleaning a cleanroom can generate many particles. To minimise contamination generated by the cleaning process the air conditioning should be fully on.
- Cleaning staff should have the same standard of clothing and gloves as the production staff.
- Cleaning must be done slower than would be the case in the home. This will minimise dispersion and ensure more efficient cleaning.
- Cleaning agents may be diluted in a bucket with distilled or deionised water, or with water as clean as can be provided.
- Bottles with spray nozzles are used to apply a cleaning agent or disinfectant. However, tests I carried out showed that they release over 1 million particles ≥ 0.5 μm with every spray. It is therefore best to cover the spray nozzle with the wiper when applying the solution. Dispensing by a hand pump is probably a better alternative.
- Cleaning or disinfectant agents used in the 'critical' area should be chosen to do the least harm to the product and be at the lowest concentration to do the job effectively.
- Diluted detergents can support microbial growth, so cleaning agents should be prepared freshly from the concentrated solution and then stored for the minimum time. Containers used for handling the diluted agent should not be left about and continually topped up, as there may be bacteria growing in the container. Containers should be thoroughly washed out after use and left to dry.

21.5.2 Cleaning methods with respect to area type

- When setting up a schedule for cleaning a room, consider the fact that horizontal surfaces, because of gravitational settling of particles, will become dirtier more quickly than vertical surfaces. Also surfaces that come into contact with people will become dirtier than those that do not. This means that walls and ceilings do not collect as many particles and require less cleaning than floors or doors. Doors will need more cleaning than walls because they are touched more often.
- Cleaning should be considered in relation to the 'critical', 'general' and 'outside' area concept. The 'critical' area is the production zone where contamination can gain direct access to the product. These

critical areas should be cleaned to the highest level. The 'general' area of the cleanroom is where contamination cannot directly contaminate the product, but it can be transferred to 'critical areas', e.g. walls, floors, etc. The cleaning there can therefore be less stringent. The 'outside' area is the materials air lock, clothes changing and other ancillary areas. The cleaning method here can be less strict, although because of the extra activity it may be necessary to do it more frequently.

- The most efficient cleaning methods should be used in the critical area, less efficient methods in the general area, and the least efficient in the outside areas. This means that the surface area that can be cleaned in a given time should be smallest in 'critical' areas and greatest in 'outside' areas. There is an overlap in the efficiency of cleaning methods but, generally speaking, the cleaning efficiency increases as follows:

  Dry vacuuming ⇒ single-bucket mopping ⇒ multiple-bucket mopping ⇒ damp wiping or, wet pick-up

- Dry vacuum cleaning in cleanrooms should not be thought of as a cleaning method, but as a pre-requisite to cleaning. It is generally used in outside and general areas and in critical areas that have a fast build-up of fibres or particles generated by the process. Cleaning methods vary, but in outside areas single-bucket mopping may be suitable. In general areas multiple-bucket mopping or wet pick-up can be used and in critical areas, damp wiping.
- Cleaning of the 'critical' areas should be done frequently. The idea that cleaning should be done only by designated cleaning staff is wrong. Personnel working in the cleanroom may be required to clean at times throughout the day, e.g. prior to the start of producing a fresh batch. Outside areas, owing to the fact that they are the furthest away from the area where the product is exposed to contamination could, if all other factors were equal, be cleaned less often. However, because of the high activity and debris accumulated in the change areas, it may be necessary to clean them on a more regular basis than other areas of

the cleanroom. 'General' areas should be cleaned at a frequency dependent on the standard of the cleanroom but can probably be done, prior to, or just after, the work period. This can be done either by the staff working in the room, or by contract cleaning staff. Where there is 24 hour working, cleaning must be done during production. This is less than satisfactory, but there may be no option. It may be possible to stop production in the surrounding area and cordon it off. This can stop people slipping on the wet floor.

21.5.3 Cleaning methods

- The cleaning process can start by removing the 'sticks and stones' with a dry vacuum. Fluff, fibres, glass splinters, etc. are removed but not small particles. It also removes sufficient soil to allow a lower concentration of detergent to be used. If the vacuum fails to lift large items they should be gathered together with a wet mop and removed.
- Cleaning should start at the areas furthest away from the exit. This ensures minimal recontamination of the surfaces. In a critical area in a unidirectional flow of air it is best to start at the point nearest the supply filters and move away from them.
- Attention should be paid to the cleanliness of the water. In 'outside' areas that are cleaned using a single bucket, it is generally accepted that the water should be changed when it becomes noticeably discoloured. If a three or two-bucket system is used in 'general' are as the water should not be controlled by discolouration but changed after a given surface area is cleaned.
- Use overlapping strokes of the wiper or mop. A cleanroom will always appear clean to the eye and it is not easy to ensure that every piece of the surface is cleaned, except by an overlapping pass method.
- If a damp wiper is used then it should be folded, and as the cleaning proceeds it should be refolded to give a clean surface. After all surfaces of the wiper are used it should be replaced.
- The area to be cleaned in a given time must be determined. Precision cleaning at the critical area is done very slowly, while, on the other hand, it should be possible to mop over an 'outside' area at a greater speed.

- If disinfectants are used in an aqueous form, it must be remembered that they do not act instantly. Disinfectants should be applied liberally to ensure that they do not dry off and should be left for at least two minutes, and preferably five minutes, to act. Alcohol, with or without bactericides, will dry quickly. This is permissible, as it partly depends on the drying of the alcohol to kill the bacteria.
- In 'critical' and sometimes 'general' cleaning, the process is sometimes completed by going over the surface with 'clean' water so that any residual surfactant or disinfectant is removed. This is especially useful with a single bucket system.
- In critical cleaning, the process can be finalised by vacuuming over the surface. This will ensure that any fibres left from wipers or mops are removed.

Figure 21.9 is a suggested method for cleaning the 'outside' and 'general' areas in a cleanroom. The method assumes that a single bucket is used, but a multiple-bucket method is best for a 'general' area.

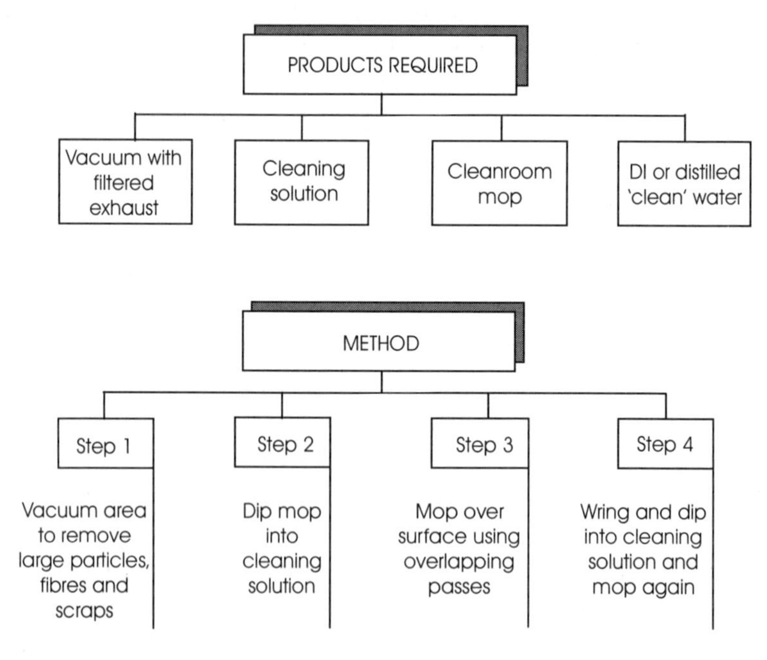

Figure 21.9 Routine cleaning of 'outside' and 'general' areas

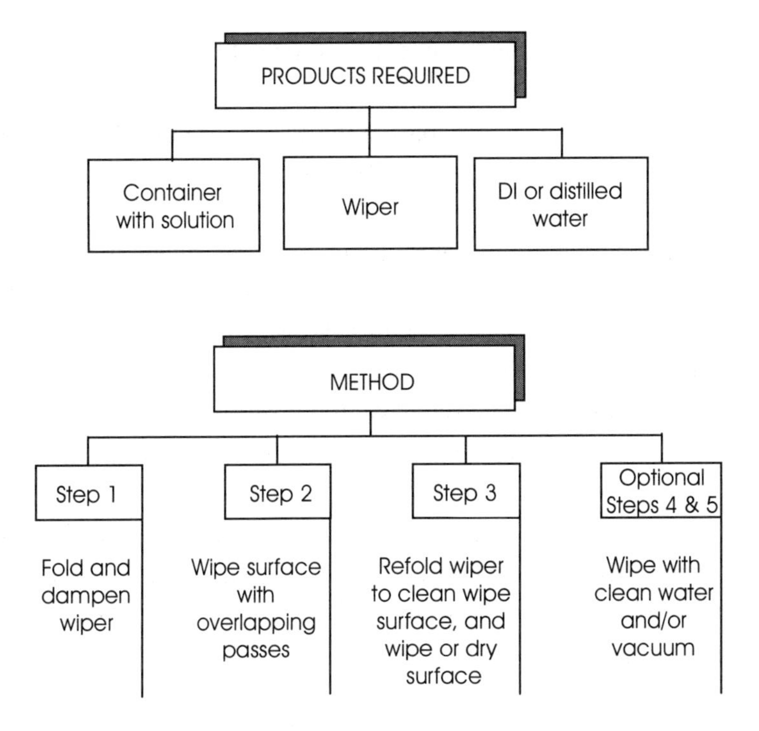

Figure 21.10 Cleaning of critical areas

Figure 21.10 shows a suggested method for 'critical' areas. A vacuum is not normally required but can be used as a preliminary step where the process disperses large numbers of fibres or large particles.

21.6 Test Methods

In the home, it is relatively simple to see if your cleaning has been unsuccessful; a look will be sufficient. In a cleanroom, dirt should never be seen, even if the cleaning has been less than successful. There are, however, a number of methods that can be used to ascertain the effectiveness of cleanroom cleaning. Some of these methods are used to establish how quickly cleanroom surfaces become soiled; this information can then be used to establish how often the surface should be cleaned. Other test methods are used to establish how much contamination is on the surface before and after cleaning, and hence, how efficient the cleaning has been. These are as follows:

1. Inspection of the cleanroom mats at the entrance to the cleanroom can sometimes be revealing. Footprints should be seen leading into the cleanroom but never out.
2. If a damp black or white wiper is drawn over a given area of cleanroom surface it is sometimes possible to concentrate the soil sufficient to indicate the amount of dirt on the surface.
3. An ultra-violet light shows up surface particles and fibres that fluoresce. For example, fibres from cleanroom garments will show up.
4. A high-intensity light shone at an acute angle to the surface, in a darkened room, shows up small particles and fibres.
5. Sticky tape can be applied to a surface and then removed. The particles stripped from the surface can be counted and sized under a microscope. ASTM E 1216-87 outlines such a method.
6. Instruments are available for measuring particles on surfaces. A sampling head is pushed over the surface and an optical particle counter measures the particles detached by the instrument.
7. A 47 mm diameter membrane holder, without the membrane support grid, can be attached to a particle counter and particles over a given area vacuumed off and counted.

Further information about test methods is available in IEST-RP-CC018.

If the efficiency of disinfection methods is required then either a contact plate or swab can be used with neutralisers against the disinfectant incorporated in the microbial media. Microbiological surface sampling methods are discussed in Chapter 14.

Acknowledgements

Figure 21.2 is reproduced by permission of Tiger-Vac. Figures 21.3 and 21.4 are reproduced by permission of Micronova Manufacturing. Figure 21.5 is reproduced by permission of Shield Medicare. Figure 21.7 is reproduced by permission of Dycem Ltd.

Index

Page numbers in italic signify references to figures, while page numbers in bold, denote references to tables.